MUSCLE RELAXANTS

CLINICAL PHARMACOLOGY

Series Editor

MURRAY WEINER

Division of Clinical Pharmacology and Toxicology
University of Cincinnati
College of Medicine
Cincinnati, Ohio

Volume 1 Nicotinic Acid: Nutrient-Cofactor-Drug, *by Murray Weiner and Jan van Eys*

Volume 2 Drugs in Central Nervous System Disorders, *edited by David C. Horwell*

Volume 3 Clinical Application of Interferons and Their Inducers, Second Edition, *edited by Dale A. Stringfellow*

Volume 4 Beta-Lactam Antibiotics for Clinical Use, *edited by Sherry F. Queener, J. Alan Webber, and Stephen W. Queener*

Volume 5 Receptor Binding in Drug Research, *edited by Robert A. O'Brien*

Volume 6 Drug Therapy in Hypertension, *edited by Jan I. M. Drayer, David T. Lowenthal, and Michael A. Weber*

Volume 7 Muscle Relaxants: Side Effects and a Rational Approach to Selection, *edited by Isaac Azar*

Volume 8 Clinical Pharmacology in the Elderly, *edited by Cameron G. Swift*

Volume 9 Anti-Inflammatory Compounds, *edited by W. R. Nigel Williamson*

MUSCLE RELAXANTS

Side Effects and a Rational Approach to Selection

edited by

Isaac Azar
Beth Israel Medical Center
New York, New York

MARCEL DEKKER, INC. New York and Basel

Library of Congress Cataloging-in-Publication Data

Muscle Relaxants: Side Effects and a Rational Approach to Selection

(Clinical pharmacology ; v. 7)
Includes index.
1. Muscle relaxants—Side effects. 2. Muscle relaxants—Toxicology. 3. Muscle relaxants—Physiological effects. I. Azar, Isaac [date] II. Series.
[DNLM: 1. Cardiovascular System—drug effects. 2. Curare-Like Agents—adverse effects. 3. Muscle Relaxants, Central—adverse effects. 4. Neuromuscular Blocking Agents—adverse effects. W1 CL764H v.7 / QV140 A244]
RM312.A38 1987 615'.77 86-24308
ISBN 0-8247-7645-3

MARCEL DEKKER, INC.
270 Madison Avenue, New York, New York 10016

Current printing (last digit):
10 9 8 7 6 5 4 3 2 1

PRINTED IN THE UNITED STATES OF AMERICA

לזכר הורי
סלמה ושמואל עזר

Dedicated to
Irene, Dan, Oren, and Gila-Anat
whose love made this possible

Series Introduction

Ever since civilized man identified curare, the arrow-tip poison, as being paralytic by blockade of the neuromuscular junction with essentially no central nervous system effect, there has been increasing interest in this mechanism to achieve clinically desirable muscular relaxation. Over the years its use has been considered for a wide variety of muscle dystonias, from acute sprains to a pharmacologic substitute for the "spasmolytic" warm packs of Sister Kenny's treatment of acute poliomyelitis in the early 1950s. A major use has been to help the anesthesiologist give the surgeon the flaccid patient he often wants.

The simple truth of the pharmacologic mechanism of curare was the basis of years of clinical use of d-tubocurarine and succinylcholine and derivatives. However, the whole truth concerning these drugs is far from simple.

In this scholarly volume, Dr. Azar has collected a body of information illustrating the frequently forgotten fact that drugs often have actions besides those that lead us to take an interest in them. Like it or not, we are obliged to pay attention to *all* the effects of the muscle relaxants, and particularly to identify those clinical situations in which these other effects are of particular importance.

Our clinical pharmacology series is designed to help both practitioner and researcher. This volume deals with muscle relaxants in a manner that is bound to improve the ability of practitioners to select the best muscle relaxant for a particular patient. It also points up the characteristics to be targeted in the search for safer and more useful muscle relaxants. It is a significant contribution to the field.

Murray Weiner, M.D.

Foreword

"Where there was sufficient data to judge, no impressive differences in death rate among several muscle relaxants were observed here. While the data are too few to permit establishment of rates for the newer agents, death has occurred in association with each, including the new succinylcholine. No pretext is made of being able to spot a curare death apart from what has been defined as an anesthesia death. The significant point is that when the muscle relaxants entered the situation, the anesthesia death rate increases nearly six-fold, from an anesthesia death rate of 1:2100 (based upon 266 anesthesia deaths) to a rate of 1:370 (based upon 118 anesthesia deaths in 44,100 patients who received curare). These data suggest that the widespread custom of using curare for many trivial purposes is not justified.

"A new observation is made here that, despite artificial respiration of a generally effective type (bag squeezing), many curare patients die of circulatory collapse. It is not, heretofore, been recognized that a common cause of death from curare is circulatory failure." (From Beecher HK and Todd DP: A study of the deaths associated with anesthesia and surgery. *Ann Surg 140*: 30, 1954.)

Considering these statements, extracted from a report of anesthetic practices in major academic institutions, it is somewhat of a miracle that the use of neuromuscular blocking agents so quickly became essential components of safe anesthetic practices. Because some of the methodology in the Beecher-Todd report was flawed, the conclusions were invalid. Nevertheless, it took some years to recognize that the use of neuromuscular blocking agents and spontaneous ventilation are incompatible. Additional years of practice and astute observations were required before ganglionic blockade and histamine release were recognized as sequelae to d-tubocurarine administration.

Succinylcholine was hailed as curare's successor and was thought to be devoid of ganglionic-blocking and histamine-releasing properties. Years of use later, the side effects complicating the use of succinylcholine were legion. They extend from causing arrhythmias, increasing intraocular pressure, causing prolonged apnea, injuring muscle membranes, causing elevated potassium levels, triggering malignant hyperpyrexic syndrome, and causing death. If succinylcholine were a new drug today, it is unlikely that the Food and Drug Administration would approve its use, given these side effects. And yet who among us would choose to practice anesthesiology without succinylcholine?

All neuromuscular blocking agents introduced to date have the potential for causing side effects. Those that produce untoward reactions at the usual clinical dosage necessary to produce surgical relaxation must be discarded. Agents that have an appropriate therapeutic and safety ratio are required. Because the most significant side effects that attend the use of muscle relaxants are those that affect the cardiovascular system, Savarese and colleagues have devised a method of determining the margin of safety of all neuromuscular blocking drugs. The newest agents available in clinical practice must now be devoid of cardiovascular side effects at doses at least three or more times that used in clinical settings. Such drugs are now available and are the standards of safe clinical practice.

But what of their reversal with atropine and neostigmine, themselves somewhat dangerous because of their effects on the cardiovascular systems? It would be best to avoid these agents;

this can be most appropriately done by monitoring neuromuscular transmission whenever muscle relaxants are used. This too should be a standard of practice as safe patient management requires it.

And what of the future? All clinicians and academicians agree that a short-acting, nondepolarizing neuromuscular blocking agent devoid of cardiovascular or other side effects would be an important contribution to patient management. The search for such a drug started with Bovet a half-century ago. Several thousand pretenders have been synthesized, studied, and abandoned. The search not only continues but is expanding dramatically, pushed by the twin forces of increasing knowledge of the chemistry involved and the demands of the marketplace. The optimists among us, and I am one, believe that such an agent will be ours by the end of this decade. But until then we must use less than perfect agents and must be attentive to their potential for causing deleterious effects in addition to their desired action. Recognizing the situation, Dr. Isaac Azar has recruited outstanding contributions from world-class scientists and clinicians and collated these in this superb text, *Muscle Relaxants: Side Effects and a Rational Approach to Selection.* It is a most important contribution, summarizing in one volume the most relevant information concerning untoward effects of this class of compounds. This book is dedicated to improving our patient's anesthetic management when muscle relaxants are used and hence represents an important contribution to the safe practice of anesthesiology.

Richard J. Kitz, M.D.
Harvard Medical School
Boston, Massachusetts

Preface

Before the introduction of curare to the practice of anesthesia in 1942, anesthesiologists resorted to the use of deep inhalation anesthesia to produce muscle relaxation and to facilitate surgery. This technique often resulted in significant cardiovascular depression and prolonged postoperative recovery. The introduction of muscle relaxants greatly enhanced the management of surgical patients and critically ill patients. The affinity of muscle relaxants for nicotinic cholinergic receptors at the neuromuscular junction makes them potent neuromuscular blockers without causing significant depression of the central nervous system.

Over the years, however, it became obvious that the administration of muscle relaxants was often accompanied by adverse and abnormal reactions. Histamine release, autonomic ganglionic blockade, potassium release, and prolonged apnea are frequently observed and, on occasion, are accompanied by morbidity and mortality.

Several groups of patients are particularly susceptible to the untoward effects of muscle relaxants. Patients with neuromuscular disorders often exhibit abnormal responses to muscle relaxants such as resistance, exaggerated response, and potassium release. The tendency of patients with muscle paralysis or extensive burns to release potassium following the administration of succinylcholine is particularly dangerous; this is occasionally followed by cardiac arrest.

Some genetic abnormalities have also been shown to cause abnormal responses to muscle relaxants. Malignant hyperthermia, a rare but potentially lethal disorder, may be triggered by succinylcholine and volatile anesthetic agents. Another genetic abnormality, atypical pseudocholinesterase, occurs in about 2.5% of the population. Unlike the normal enzyme, atypical pseudocholinesterase metabolizes succinylcholine poorly and so the usual doses of succinylcholine cause prolonged paralysis in these patients.

A large segment of our patient population has compromised kidney and liver functions. Accordingly, the response of these patients to muscle relaxants is often exaggerated and prolonged. This is of particular importance in elderly and in critically ill patients. In recent years much progress has been made through the study of the pharmacodynamics and the pharmacokinetics of different muscle relaxants, and a more rational approach to the selection of a muscle relaxant for a particular patient is now possible. Additionally, new intermediate-acting muscle relaxants with minimal cardiovascular effects have been introduced. We can now select a muscle relaxant that suits the particular needs of the individual patient and significantly reduces the danger of adverse and abnormal reactions.

This textbook is a compilation of information on adverse and abnormal reactions to muscle relaxants. It should be useful to anesthesiologists, critical care physicians, and other medical specialists who use muscle relaxants in their practice. The editor and authors of this book hope that it will contribute to the improved care of patients treated with muscle relaxants.

The editor gratefully acknowledges the editorial assistance of Terry Torchinsky and of Erwin Lear, M.D., and the pleasant and efficient working relationship with Paul Dolgert and Carol S. Carol of Marcel Dekker, Inc. Special thanks go to Irene Tkaczuk and Maria Herasimchuk for expert preparation of the manuscript.

Isaac Azar, M.D

Contents

Contributors

Isaac Azar, M.D. Department of Anesthesiology, Beth Israel Medical Center, New York, New York

Jeffrey E. Fletcher, Ph.D. Department of Anesthesiology, Hahnemann University School of Medicine, Philadelphia, Pennsylvania

*David R. Goldhill, M.B.B.S.** Department of Anaesthesia, Harvard Medical School, and Department of Anesthesia, Shriners Burn Institute, Boston, Massachusetts

Nishan G. Goudsouzian, M.D. Department of Anaesthesia, Harvard Medical School, and Department of Anesthesia, Massachusetts General Hospital, Boston, Massachusetts

**Present affiliation*: The London Hospital, London, England

J. A. Jeevendra Martyn, M.D. Department of Anesthesia, Shriners Burn Institute, and Department of Anesthesia, Massachusetts General Hospital, Boston, Massachusetts

Carol B. Pantuck Department of Anesthesiology, College of Physicians and Surgeons, Columbia University, New York, New York

Eugene J. Pantuck, M.D. Department of Anesthesiology, College of Physicians and Surgeons, Columbia University, New York, New York

Henry Rosenberg, M.D. Department of Anesthesiology, Hahnemann University School of Medicine, Philadelphia, Pennsylvania

Stephen M. Rupp, M.D. Department of Anesthesia, University of California, San Francisco, San Francisco, California

John J. Savarese, M.D. Department of Anaesthesia, Harvard Medical School, and Department of Anesthesia, Massachusetts General Hospital, Boston, Massachusetts

*Ralph P. F. Scott, M.B.Ch.B., F.F.A.R.C.C.** Department of Anaesthesia, Harvard Medical School, and Department of Anesthesia, Massachusetts General Hospital, Boston, Massachusetts

---

**Present affiliation*: Southampton General Hospital, Southampton, England

MUSCLE RELAXANTS

1
Autonomic Responses to Muscle Relaxants

RALPH P. F. SCOTT* and JOHN J. SAVARESE
Harvard Medical School, and Massachusetts General Hospital, Boston, Massachusetts

**Present affiliation*: Southampton General Hospital, Southampton, England

I. INTRODUCTION

The use of neuromuscular-blocking agents has produced a tremendous advance in facilitating surgical technique. These drugs however are not entirely without hazard, and a variety of studies over the years have highlighted deficiencies common to all the well-established muscle relaxants in current use. In particular, they lack the degree of specificity that the ideal blocking agent should show for the neuromuscular junction, especially with respect to freedom from cardiovascular side effects. These cardiovascular effects are generally due to either stimulation or inhibition of peripheral autonomic sites, to increases in serum potassium levels secondary to motor end plate depolarization, or to the release of histamine and possibly other vasoactive substances from vascular mast cells. The release of histamine has been discussed in Chapter 2 in this book, and for the purpose of this chapter, the authors will confine themselves to describing the autonomic effects of both nondepolarizing and depolarizing neuromuscular-blocking agents.

At present the most commonly used neuromuscular-blocking agents in anesthetic practice in the United States are succinylcholine, d-tubocurarine, metocurine, and pancuronium. A careful examination of the advantages and disadvantages of these blockers leads to the conclusion that a short-acting nondepolarizing muscle relaxant to replace succinylcholine and a long-acting muscle relaxant without cardiovascular side effects to replace pancuronium would provide significant improvements.

As the mode of action of these drugs has become better understood, the possibility of designing specific compounds that meet the demands of the clinician has become more realistic. The accumulated knowledge in the field of neuromuscular blockade is now such that medicinal chemists are able to produce effective neuromuscular-blocking agents more predictably with less reliance on chance than is the case with any other class of drugs. Consequently, most kinds of unwanted activity can be avoided altogether by appropriate molecular design and any new compounds that do happen to produce unwanted effects can often be discarded at an early state in preclinical testing.

The development of atracurium and vecuronium has marked an exciting stage in the production of agents with cardiovascular stability. However, both drugs fall into the intermediate-duration class, and research is continuing to find agents with similar cardiovascular stability but with shorter and longer durations of action.

II. PHARMACOLOGY OF CHOLINOCEPTIVE SITES

In order to understand the autonomic responses to muscle relaxants it is important to have a working knowledge of the autonomic nervous system and in particular the possible sites of interaction between muscle relaxants and cholinoceptors.

Acetylcholine acts on muscarinic and nicotinic receptors (Table 1). Muscarinic receptors are present in various smooth muscles, cardiac muscles, and exocrine glands. They are termed muscarinic because muscarine, a quarternary amine alkaloid, has actions similar to those of acetylcholine at the sites indicated. The muscarinic receptor is blocked by atropine and related drugs.

The nicotinic receptors of acetylcholine are located in autonomic ganglia and at the skeletal neuromuscular junction. They are termed nicotinic because nicotine also acts on these

Table 1 Cholinoceptive Sites

Site	Activator or substrates	Inhibitor
Nicotinic receptors	Nicotine, tetramethylammonium	d-Tubocurarine
neuromuscular junction	Succinylcholine, decamethonium	All nondepolarizing neuromuscular block agents
autonomic ganglia	Dimethylphenylpiperazinium	Hexamethonium, d-tubocurarine
Muscarinic receptors (bowel, bladder bronchi, sinus node of the heart, pupillary sphincter)	Muscarine	Atropine, gallamine, pancuronium
Esteratic receptors		
active site of acetylcholinesterase	Acetylcholine, methacholine	Neostigmine, pyridostigmine, benzoquinonium
active site of plasmacholinesterase	Benzoylcholine, butyrylcholine, succinylcholine	Hexaflurenium, tetrahydrodaminocrine, pancuronium

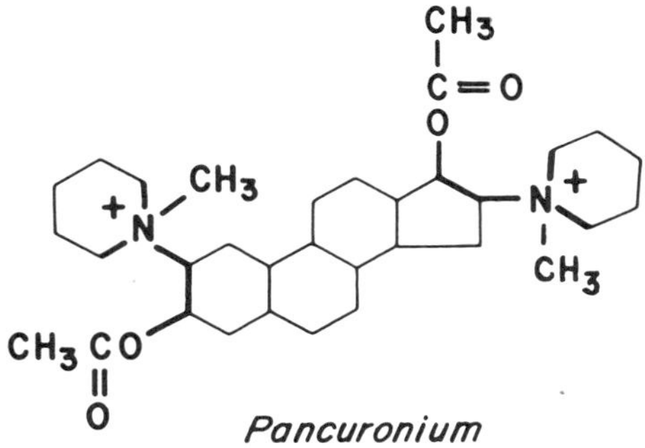

Pancuronium

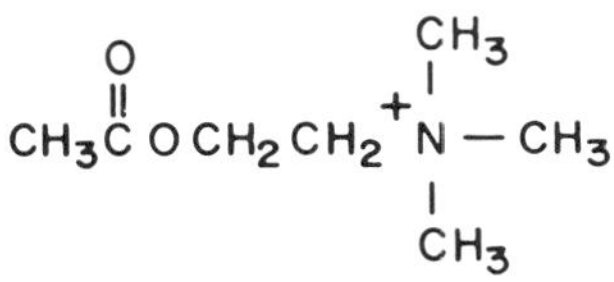

Acetylcholine

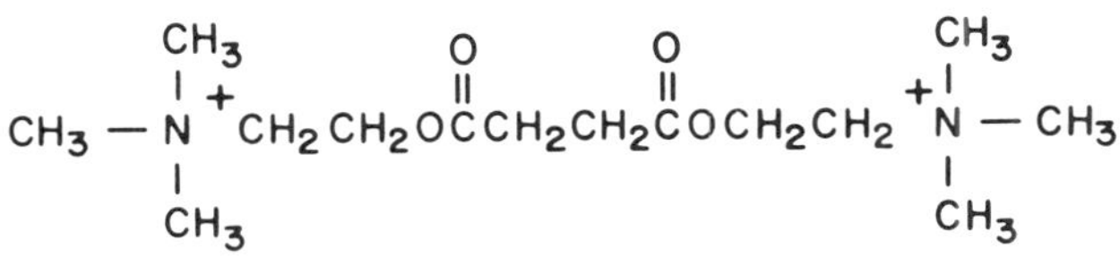

Succinylcholine
(diacetylcholine)

Figure 1 Structural relationship of acetylcholine to two neuromuscular-blocking agents. Succinylcholine (diacetylcholine) is simply two molecules of acetylcholine linked through the acetate methyl groups. Pancuronium may be viewed as two acetylcholinelike fragments (outlined in dark print) properly orientated conformationally on a bulky rigid inflexible steroid nucleus.

receptors. However, the nicotinic receptors in autonomic ganglia and in skeletal muscle are not identical. The effect of acetylcholine on autonomic ganglia is blocked by hexamethonium, whereas the skeletal neuromuscular junction is blocked by d-tubocurarine and related compounds.

Further cholinoceptive sites are found on the esteratic receptors of acetylcholinesterase and plasma cholinesterase.

A partial isolation of the cholinergic receptor has been achieved as a result of studies on some snake venoms that combine irreversibly with such receptors. It has been shown that alpha-bungarotoxin exerts a postsynaptic-blocking action similar to that of d-tubocurarine except that it is irreversible (1). The toxin can be labeled radioactively, and it serves admirably for the isolation and study of some cholinergic receptors.

Crystallographic analysis of acetylcholine and related agonists provides a tentative answer to the nature of the cholinergic receptor. Acetylcholine is a flexible molecule and rotation is possible at two different bonds (see Fig. 1). Muscarinic and nicotinic drugs differ from acetylcholine in the degree of rotation at the sites of torsion. Thus, acetylcholine has both muscarinic and nicotinic effects, whereas the purely muscarinic or nicotinic congeners have constraints imposed on them by conformational factors.

In order for neuromuscular-blocking agents to interact with the recognition sites of the cholinoceptors at the neuromuscular junction, the drugs must bear some chemical relationship to acetylcholine. Consequently, there is a possibility that they might compete with or mimic acetylcholine at other sites (e.g., cholinesterase, nicotinic autonomic ganglionic receptors, and muscarinic receptors).

III. INTERACTION OF NEUROMUSCULAR-BLOCKING AGENTS AT DIFFERENT CHOLINOCEPTIVE SITES

A. Autonomic Ganglia

d-Tubocurarine (Fig. 2) blocks ganglionic nicotinic receptors and produces some ganglionic blockade in a dose range slightly greater than that required to produce neuromuscular blockade. It may

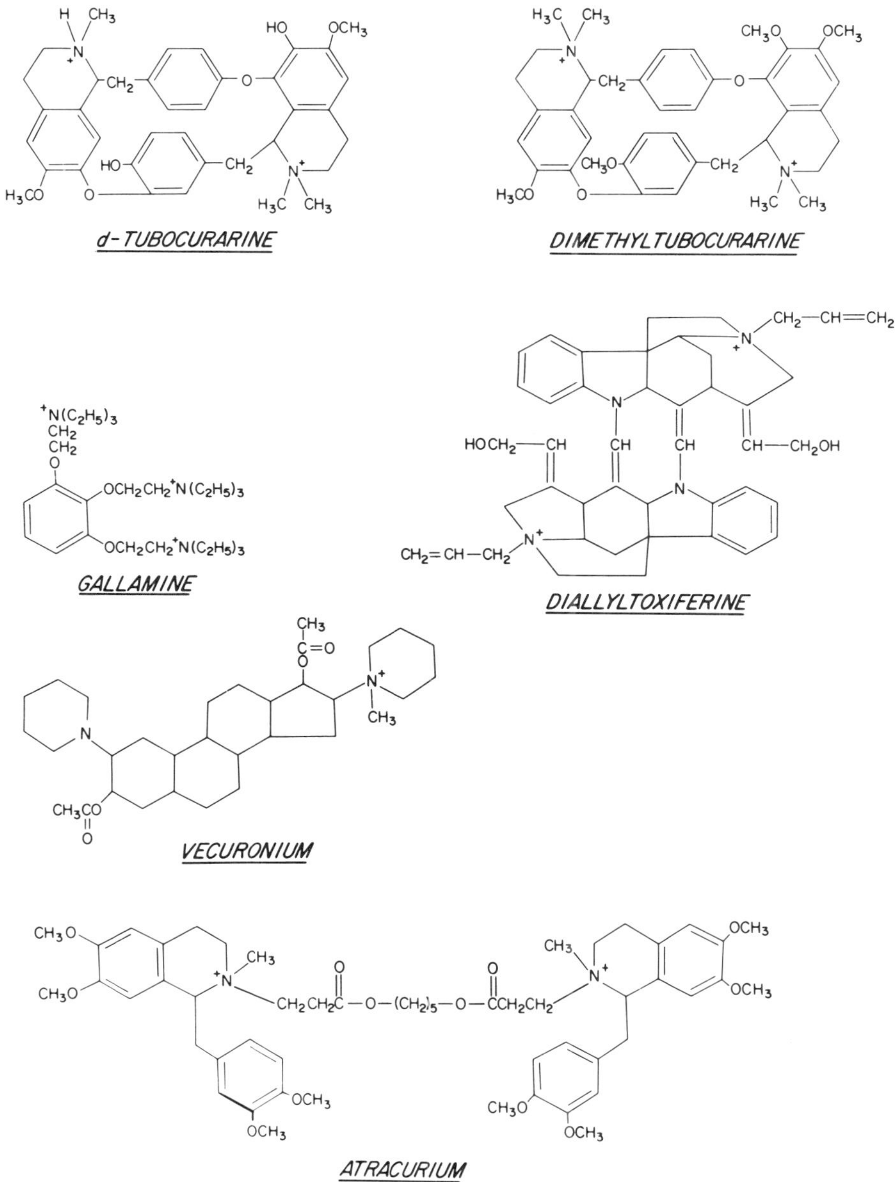

Figure 2 The chemical structure of some common nondepolarizing neuromuscular-blocking agents.

have a slightly more powerful action on parasympathetic than on sympathetic ganglia (2). Autonomic reflexes arising in the course of surgical operations may be impaired by this ganglion-blocking action (3), and this action may contribute to hypotension (4). However, there is evidence suggesting that the role of ganglionic blockade in the hypotensive action of d-tubocurarine is possibly less important than its ability to release histamine (5). Metocurine and alcuronium are weaker ganglion blockers, and other neuromuscular-blocking drugs (gallamine, pancuronium, atracurium, and vecuronium) have no ganglion-blocking activity in the doses used clinically. Succinylcholine has a weak ganglion-stimulant action (6), which may be of some importance.

B. Muscarinic Receptors

By definition, all muscarinic receptors are stimulated by muscarine and are blocked by atropine. However, evidence has accumulated in recent years that these receptors are probably not a homogeneous group, and that they may differ with respect to their interactions with other agonists and antagonists. Figure 3 is a diagrammatic representation of the main components of the autonomic nervous system with respect to the heart. For the purpose of the diagram, these muscarinic receptors have been labeled M_1, M_2, and M_3 receptors, but this is not a strict classification and is probably an over simplification (7).

The first indication that muscarinic receptors may not all be identical in character came from the work of Riker and Wescoe (8), who showed that gallamine, although generally free from atropinelike activity in smooth muscle, nevertheless blocked muscarinic receptors in the cat heart and consequently inhibited the cardiac vagus. In Figure 3, these cardiac muscarinic receptors are included in the M_2 group to distinguish them from the more usual type, labeled M_1. Other workers have since shown that pancuronium (9), fazadinium (10), alcuronium (11), and stercuronium (12) also block cardiac muscarinic receptors in doses approximating those required to cause muscle relaxation. d-Tubocurarine, metocurine, vecuronium, and atracurium block cardiac muscarinic receptors and other muscarinic receptors only in doses that greatly exceed the neuromuscular-blocking dose (13–15).

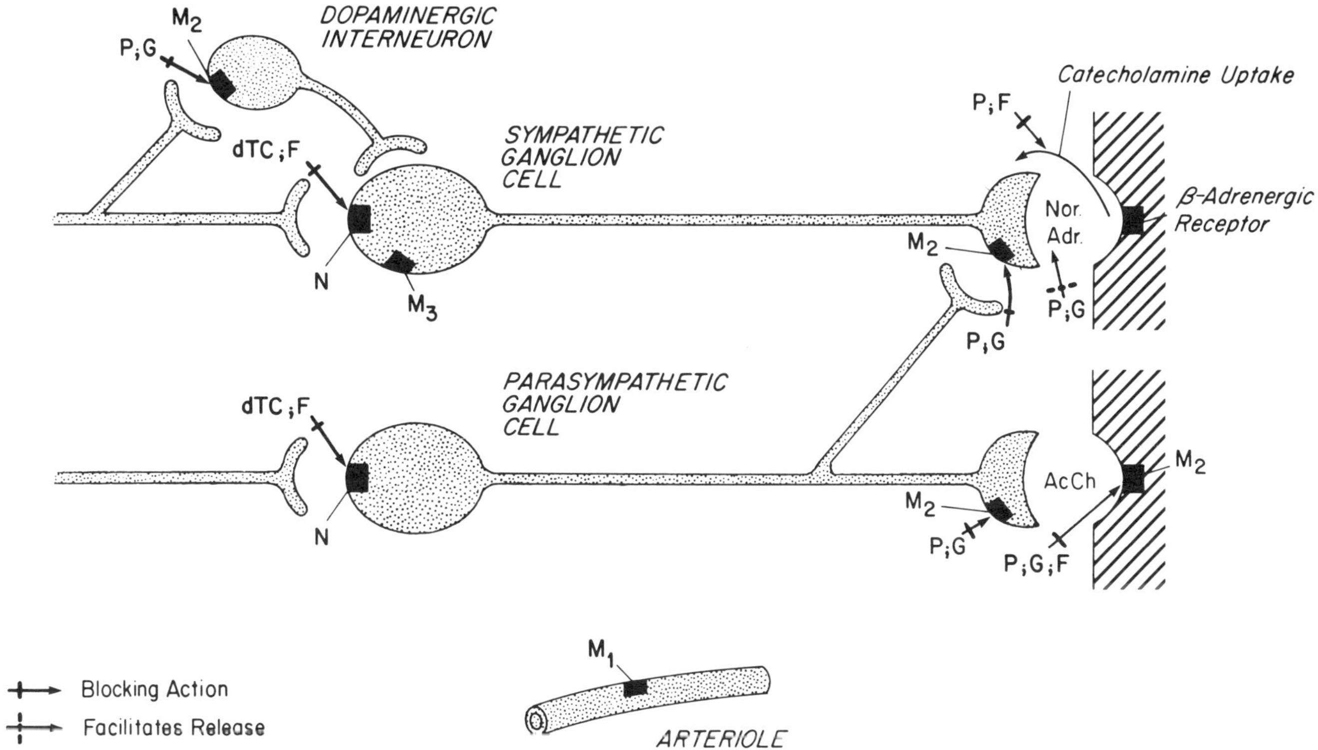

Figure 3 Diagrammatic representation of the autonomic nervous system with respect to the heart, and sites of action of some neuromuscular-blocking drugs on this system. The muscarinic receptors have been divided into three subclasses (M_1, M_2, M_3). Abbreviations: N, nicotinic receptor; P, pancuronium; G, gallamine; F, fazadinium; dTC, d-Tubocurarine.

Arterioles also have muscarinic receptors, but these receptors are not innervated. They resemble mostly noncardiac muscarinic receptors in their agonist and antagonist activity and are labeled M_1 in Figure 3. The vasodepressor response to methacholine, although blocked by atropine, is not affected by pancuronium, showing that the muscarinic receptors involved in the arterioles are not the same type as those in the sinoatrial node.

Experiments have shown that cardiac muscarinic receptors are not the only muscarinic receptors that are blocked by certain neuromuscular-blocking drugs. Stimulation of the vagus has been shown to reduce the release of norepinephrine from concomitently stimulated sympathetic nerves to the heart (16). It is therefore believed that vagal nerve terminals impinge not only upon the nodal and atrial cells of the heart but also on the sympathetic nerve endings where they act to inhibit the release of norepinephrine. The cholinoceptors on the sympathetic nerve endings are of the muscarinic type, and there is indirect evidence that they are blocked by gallamine and pancuronium (17), but much less effectively by vecuronium. This effect would enhance the tachycardia arising from blockade of the cardiac muscarinic receptors. Because the muscarinic receptors on the sympathetic terminals resemble the cardiac muscarinic receptors in being blocked by gallamine and pancuronium, they have been both labeled M_2, but the evidence of similarity is no stronger than this.

Another location of muscarinic receptors that are blocked by pancuronium and gallamine, and are therefore indicated as M_2 receptors in Figure 3, is on the small dopaminergic interneurons on sympathetic ganglia. These cells are activated through muscarinic receptors stimulated by acetylcholine that is released from collaterals of the preganglionic cholinergic fibers. Dopamine release from these cells onto the postganglionic neurons hyperpolarizes them and therefore suppresses ganglionic transmission (18). These cholinoceptors may also be blocked by pancuronium and gallamine and may therefore facilitate transmission through the ganglia by inactivating the inhibitory-modulating influence of the dopaminergic cell loop (19).

Transmission through sympathetic ganglia is mediated by acetylcholine acting on nicotinic receptors. There are, however, muscarinic cholinoceptors present on sympathetic ganglia whose physiological function is as yet unknown. These are labeled M_3

receptors in Figure 3. They differ from those labeled M_2 in that they are not blocked by gallamine or pancuronium, and they differ from those labeled M_1 (and M_2) in that they are especially sensitive to certain unusual muscarinic agonists (20).

It should be noted that gallamine causes norepinephrine release in guinea pig and cat atria and in anesthetized cats by a mechanism that may be quite independent of muscarinic blockade (21). Similarly, very large concentrations of pancuronium produce norepinephrine release in isolated guinea pig atria under conditions in which parasympathetic block could not be involved (22).

Pancuronium and fazadinium have been shown to block norepinephrine reuptake into sympathetic nerve endings both in cardiac muscle and in smooth muscle in guinea pigs and rats (22–24).

In the cat, the main mechanism through which certain neuromuscular-blocking drugs depress cardiovagal activity is by blocking the postjunctional muscarinic cholinoceptors as described above. However, other workers have calculated that the concentrations of pancuronium and gallamine that block responses to postjunctional vagal stimulation are too low to assert significant blocking action on the postjunctional muscarinic receptors, and they conclude that the main site of action of these two drugs in blocking the guinea pig cardiac vagus is on the postganglionic nerve terminals (25).

It can be concluded from the foregoing discussion that a combination of any of the above actions of gallamine, pancuronium, and fazadinium may account for the cardiovascular effects on these drugs. There is considerable species difference with regard to the relative importance of these effects. It is not known which effect is most predominant in man, but it is likely that the relative importance varies from patient to patient according to such factors as the preexisting autonomic balance, the type of premedication given, the anesthetic used, and any concurrent drug therapy.

C. Cholinesterase Inhibition

In practice, the anticholinesterase activities of only two neuromuscular blockers are relevant in relation to the extracellular fluid concentrations that produce neuromuscular blockade. These are the antiacetylcholinesterase action of benzoquinonium and the antibutyrylcholinesterase action of pancuronium. The anticholinesterase-inhibiting action of benzoquinonium is a serious disadvantage, not only because of the autonomic side effects to which it gives rise but also because so much of the enzyme is inhibited that anticholinesterase agents have little or no ability to reverse its neuromuscular-blocking action. This led to its withdrawal as a neuromuscular-blocking agent.

The physiological function of plasma butyrylcholinesterase is unknown, and inhibition of this enzyme by pancuronium is therefore of little consequence in practical terms.

IV. STRUCTURE-ACTIVITY RELATIONSHIPS

The natural transmitter at the neuromuscular junction, acetylcholine, has a positively charged ammonium group which is attracted to the negatively charged cholinergic receptor site. This feature is also common to the neuromuscular-blocking drugs, which contain at least one quarternary ammonium group (Figs. 1 and 2).

The neuromuscular-blocking agents show certain structural similarities to acetylcholine. Succinylcholine is essentially two molecules of acetylcholine linked through the acetate methyl groups.

Depolarizing agents such as succinylcholine generally stimulate nicotinic and muscarinic receptors in imitation of the role of acetylcholine. The depolarizing action of succinylcholine is due to the presence in the molecule of the trimethyl ammonium group and the carboxyl groups in a linear flexible chain (Fig. 1). The separation of the terminal functions from the carboxyl groups by a distance of 4.5 angstroms, as occurs with acetylcholine, also contributes to the agonist (depolarizing) action of succinylcholine (26). Removal of the carboxyl groups of succinylcholine results in decamethonium, which has much weaker autonomic-stimulating properties than succinylcholine (27).

The shape and flexibility of the molecule is also important. Most agonists such as succinylcholine are flexible, long, and slender. Bulky molecules such as pancuronium with a rigid ring system cannot activate or stimulate the receptors themselves but instead block the acetylcholine and receptor reaction, and so produce a nondepolarizing block by competitive receptor inhibition.

d-Tubocurarine (Fig. 2) has now been shown to have only one quarternary ammonium group and a tertiary amine group in equilibrium with a proton at physiological pH (28). In general, bisquarternary compounds do not possess strong ganglion-blocking or histamine-releasing properties. Methylation of d-tubocurarine to produce metocurine or dimethyl tubocurarine (a bisquarternary compound) reduces the histamine-releasing and ganglion-blocking activities associated with d-tubocurarine and results in a muscle relaxant that is three times less potent than d-tubocurarine in blocking sympathetic and parasympathetic ganglia (11,13).

Gallamine (a trisquarternary compound) has marked vagolytic properties, probably owing to the presence of three positively charged nitrogen atoms (8,11).

Increasing knowledge of the pharmacology of amino steroids resulted in the development of vecuronium (see Figs. 1 and 2). Chemically, vecuronium is simply pancuronium without the quarternary methyl group in the 2-piperidino substitution. This seemingly minor chemical difference is responsible for all the considerable pharmacological differences between vecuronium and pancuronium. The absence of this methyl group reduces the acetylcholinelike characteristics of the molecule in the area of ring A of the steroidal nucleus, thereby lessening the vagolytic property without loss of neuromuscular-blocking activity. The ring D substituents are retained intact from pancuronium and are responsible for high neuromuscular-blocking potency but not for the vagolytic effect.

V. DEMONSTRATION OF AUTONOMIC EFFECTS OF NEUROMUSCULAR-BLOCKING AGENTS IN WHOLE ANIMALS

There are no appropriate means for testing the autonomic effects of relaxants in man, and most of our knowledge of these actions is derived from experiments performed in isolated organ systems or in whole animals such as the cat.

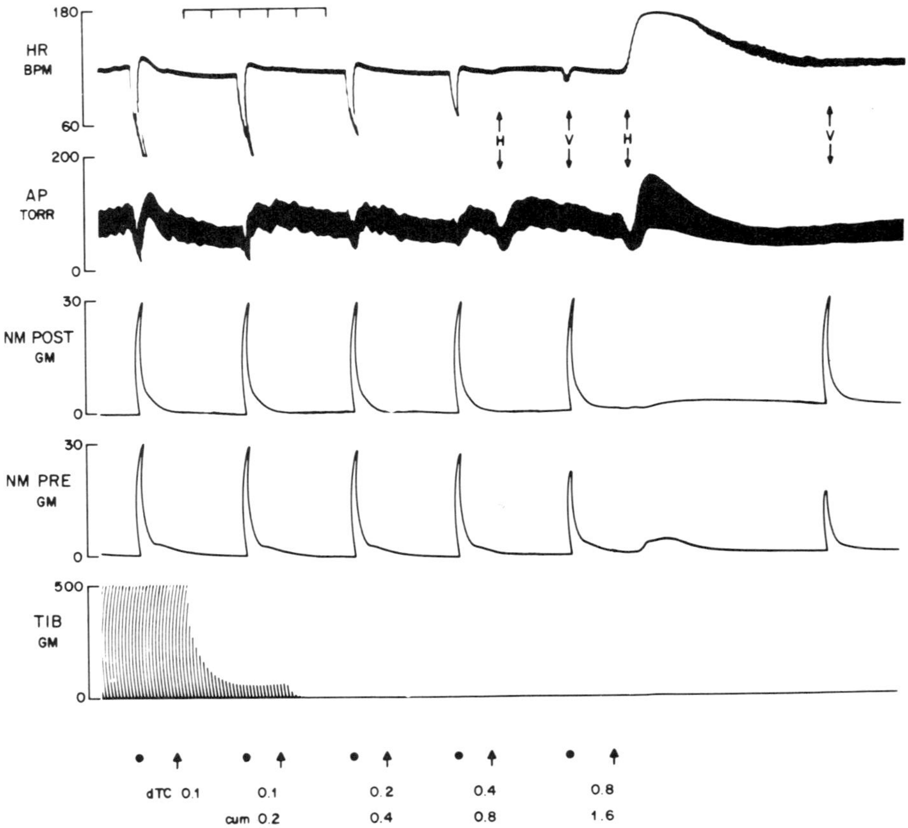

Figure 4 Simultaneous recording of autonomic and neuromuscular function in a cat anesthetized with chloralase. Recordings are (top to bottom) of heart rate, femoral arterial pressure, contractions of the left and right nictitating membranes elicited preganglionically and postganglionically, and tibialis anterior muscle twitch. At times indicated by dots below the graphs, stimulation of the right vagus nerve and both sympathetic trunks (left postganglionically and right preganglionically) was applied at 20 Hz for 10 sec. At times indicated by arrows below graphs, d-tubocurarine in doses indicated (mg/kg) was given IV. Lower figures indicate cumulative dosage. Note that vagal response (bradycardia and hypotension), ganglionic response (preganglionically stimulated nictitating membrame), and neuromuscular response are all inhibited at a cumulative dose of 0.8–1.6 mg/kg. Marker H between the upper two graphs indicates cardiovascular changes suggestive of histamine release. Marker V indicates points of vagal stimulation with little or no response.

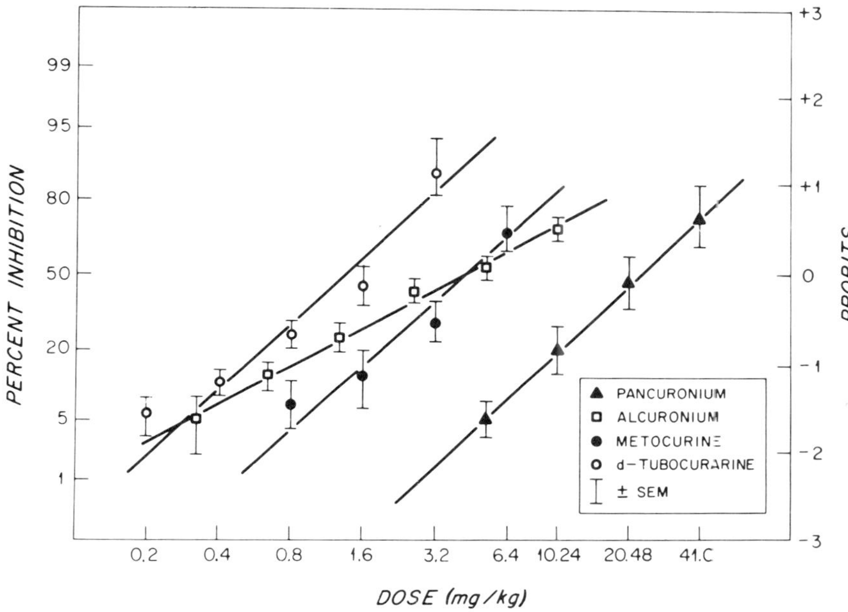

Figure 5 Dose-response curves for sympathetic inhibition by some nondepolarizing relaxants in the cat.

In the cat, measurement of neuromuscular and autonomic functions may be accomplished simultaneously. Neuromuscular function is assayed by recording the twitch response of the tibialis anterior muscle (or other appropriate muscle) evoked indirectly by the sciatic or peroneal nerve.

Vagal function is measured by quantitation of bradycardia and hypotension elicited by stimulation of the nerve. Sympathetic ganglionic responses are assayed by preganglionic stimulation of the sympathetic trunk central to the superior cervical ganglion and recording the evoked contraction of the nictitating membrane (see Fig. 4). From this information dose-response curves may be constructed for individual muscle relaxants (Fig. 5).

Table 2 Autonomic Margin of Safety of Nondepolarizing Relaxants in Man

Drug	Neuromuscular block[a]	Autonomic margin of safety		Margin of safety for histamine release
		Ganglion block	Vagal block	
d-Tubocurarine	0.51	2.94	0.59	1
Metocurine	0.28	18.6	2.86	2
Pancuronium	0.07	328.6	2.86	High
Alcuronium	0.25	18.0	1.84	High
Vecuronium	0.056	89.2	40.6	High
Atracurium	0.28	35.7	8.7	3

[a]ED_{95} in humans (mg/kg).

$$\text{Autonomic margin of safety} = \frac{ED_{50} \text{ for autonomic inhibition in the cat}}{ED_{95} \text{ for neuromuscular block in man}}$$

$$\text{Margin of safety for histamine release} = \frac{ED_{50} \text{ for histamine release in man}}{ED_{95} \text{ for neuromuscular block in man}}$$

VI. MARGIN OF SAFETY

The separation of neuromuscular-blocking action from autonomic effects can be described for each drug as its autonomic margin of safety. This indicates the number of multiples of a dose of relaxant producing 95% neuromuscular blockade that must be administered in order to produce side effects. The higher the autonomic margin of safety, the lower the probability of occurrence of a side effect. The following quotations are used:

$$\frac{\text{ED}_{50}\ \text{(ganglion block)}}{\text{ED}_{95}\ \text{(neuromuscular block)}}$$

$$\frac{\text{ED}_{50}\ \text{(cardiac vagal block}}{\text{ED}_{95}\ \text{(neuromuscular block)}}$$

Calculation of autonomic margins of safety for neuromuscular blocking drugs in man is not possible because suitable methods for quantitating autonomic responses in man are not available. There is considerable indication, however, that when a neuromuscular-blocking agent produces an autonomic effect in the cat within or near the neuromuscular dose range, the neuromuscular blockade in man will be accompanied by cardiovascular changes corresponding to those autonomic actions (see Table 2).

The ED_{95} for neuromuscular block for some of the nondepolarizing relaxants in man under nitrous oxide has been determined. These values together with the ED_{50} for ganglion and vagal block derived in the cat (since it cannot be determined in man) were used to calculate the values in Table 2.

VII. AUTONOMIC ACTIONS OF INDIVIDUAL MUSCLE RELAXANTS AND THEIR CIRCULATORY EFFECTS UNDER GENERAL ANESTHESIA

A. d-Tubocurarine

d-Tubocurarine inhibits both sympathetic and parasympathetic function at a dose range close to amounts necessary to block neuromuscular transmission (Fig. 6). This is the classic nicotinic ganglion-blocking effect of d-tubocurarine easily demonstrable in the cat (Fig. 4) (or dog) (11,29) (Table 3).

Table 3 Effects of 100%-Blocking Dose of Nondepolarizing Muscle Relaxants in Man Under Halothane Anesthesia

	Ganglion block	(Muscarinic) vagal block	Histamine release	Under anesthesia			
				SVR	COP	BP	HR
Tubocurarine	**	—	***	↓	↓	↓	—
Metocurine	*	—	**	↓	—	↓	—
Pancuronium	—	**	—	—	↑	↑	↑
Gallamine	—	***	—	—	↑	↑	↑
Alcuronium	*	*	—	↓	↑	↓	↑
Fazadinium	**	**	—	↓	↑	↓	↑
Vecuronium	—	—	—	—	—	—	—
Atracurium	—	—	—	—	—	—	—

Abbreviations: SVR, systemic vascular resistance; COP, cardiac output; BP, blood pressure (mean arterial pressure); HR, heart rate. Mild, *; moderate, **; significant, ***.

Vagal blockade by d-tubocurarine occurs at parasympathetic ganglia. The bradycardic response to direct muscarinic receptor activators such as methacholine is not inhibited, but bradycardia produced by stimulation of the vagus nerve is prevented (11,29). In the absence of histamine release, d-tubocurarine does not generally produce clinically important changes in heart rate, although it probably favors a slight bradycardia during maintenance of anesthesia. The cardiovascular effect of d-tubocurarine is due to its ganglion-blocking and histamine-releasing properties alone or in combination. The relative importance of ganglion blockade by d-tubocurarine is not entirely clear. Hypotension secondary to d-tubocurarine is rarely accompanied by dilatation of the pupil, and it is often associated with transient erythema and tachycardia, which are manifestations of systemic histamine release. The histamine-releasing effects of d-tubocurarine are discussed further in Chapter 2.

The ganglion-blocking and histamine-releasing actions of d-tubocurarine produce a fall in peripheral resistance (30). If no important change in heart rate occurs, the cardiac output may fall, particularly in the presence of an anesthetic technique that includes a myocardial depressant anesthetic vapor.

In the absence of significant myocardial depression, e.g., under nitrous oxide narcotic anesthesia, stroke volume may increase owing to improved ventricular emptying, and there may be little or no fall in cardiac output despite the occurrence of moderate hypotension.

A negative inotropic action of d-tubocurarine originally attributed to the preservative (32) has been disproved (33).

B. Metocurine

Metocurine may also be shown to block sympathetic and parasympathetic ganglia in the same manner as its parent compound, d-tubocurarine (29). It is however some three times less potent than d-tubocurarine in this respect (29). Metocurine is also a more potent neuromuscular-blocking agent than d-tubocurarine, so that its neuromuscular-blocking action is separated by a wide dose range from its autonomic effects (11). In the dog, only at eight times the ED_{95} did metocurine produce hemodynamic changes similar

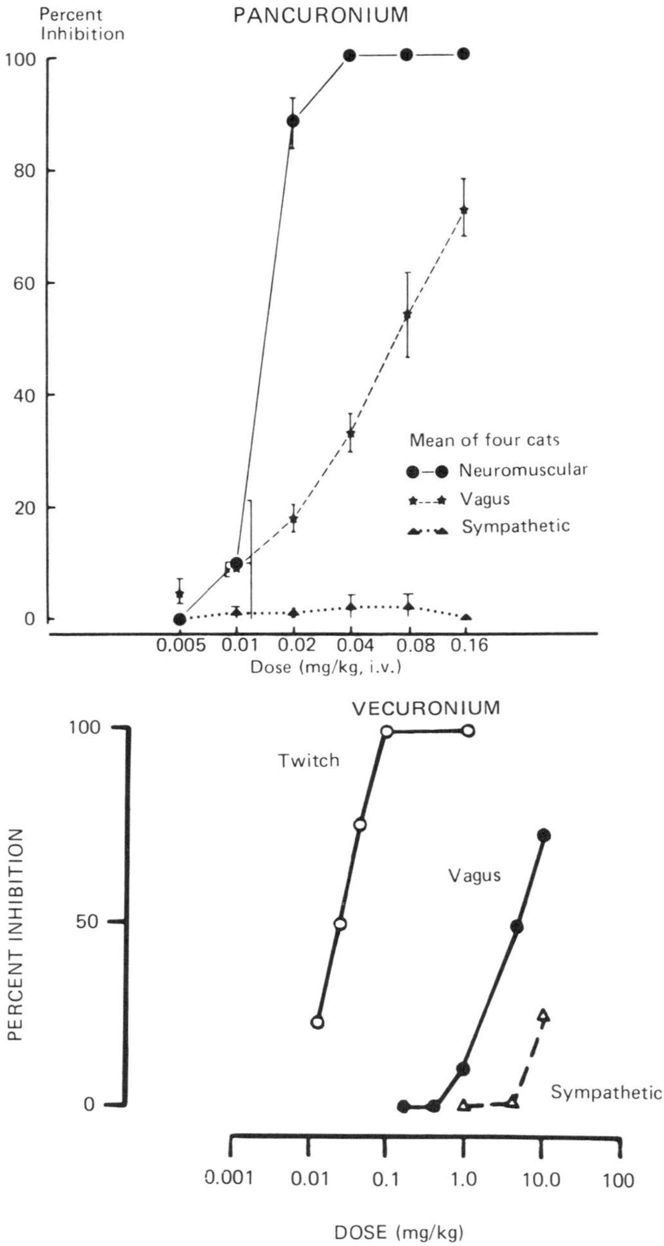

Figure 6 Dose-response curves for neuromuscular and autonomic function inhibition in cats following pancuronium, d-Tubocurarine, vecuronium (bottom left), and in monkeys following atracurium (bottom right). Note that vecuronium and atracurium cause

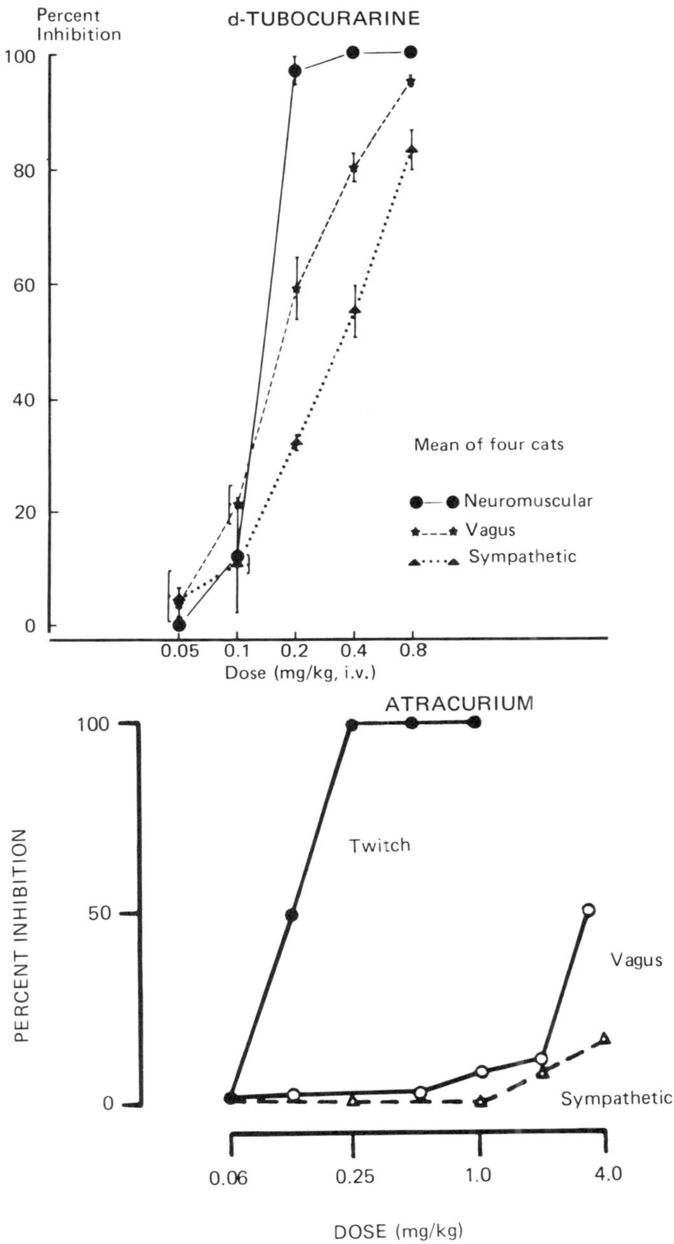

insignificant autonomic inhibition at doses considerably in excess of that required to produce 100% depression of the single twitch. (Data modified from Refs. 15 and 36.)

to those observed with d-tubocurarine at ED_{95}. The safety margin in the dog is eight times greater (34).

Brief (5–15 min) increases in heart rate may result when large bolus doses of metocurine (0.4 mg/kg or more) are given rapidly. Heart rate increases in this situation are probably manifestations of systemic histamine release by this drug.

In the absence of histamine release, metocurine does not produce clinically important chances in heart rate, although a slight bradycardia may occur during maintenance of anesthesia.

Metocurine may also produce clinical hypotension, but the incidence and severity of this side effect are probably much less than in the case of d-tubocurarine (35). In healthy patients under nitrous narcotic anesthesia, metocurine, 0.4 mg/kg, given as a rapid bolus produced an average 7% fall in mean arterial pressure. This hypotensive effect was considered to be due to histamine release in 33% of those who received this high dose (an amount more than adequate for tracheal intubation) (35). When administered more slowly (36) and to sicker patients (37) in other studies, significant cardiovascular changes have not been noted.

There is little change in cardiac output in normal man under halothane anesthesia when doses of 0.2 mg/kg are administered (38).

C. Pancuronium

The possible cardiac actions of pancuronium have already been outlined. Pancuronium has an atropinelike effect that is limited to cardiac muscarinic receptors (9,11). Experimentally, the bradycardia due to vagal stimulation or secondary to acetylcholine or methacholine is blocked (11) (Fig. 6). Increased serum catecholamine levels in humans have been measured after administration of pancuronium (39). Studies in dogs suggest a tyraminelike release of catecholamines in adrenergic nerve endings by pancuronium, i.e., an indirect sympathomimetic effect.

Workers have also noted an inhibition of neuronal uptake of norepinephrine by pancuronium in the rat (24).

Pancuronium generally produces less dramatic increases in heart rate than gallamine (40,41), and the tachycardia has not been shown to be dose dependent in humans but is inversely related to the control heart rate. The vagolytic effect of pancuronium is probably weak within the dose range required for clinical neuromuscular blockade and usually results in heart rates of 70-90 beats/minute in the average patient. Marked tachycardia may occur in a small percentage of patients. This unexpected response may be due to its indirect sympathomimetic action.

A rise in arterial pressure of 10-20 mmHg following the administration of pancuronium (30) is common, particularly under nitrous oxide narcotic anesthesia in the absence of potent anesthetic vapors. The increased heart rate resulting in an increase in cardiac output in the absence of any fall in peripheral resistance is the probable mechanism involved. Some workers have suggested that pancuronium has a weak inotropic effect on cardiac muscle (42). However, other studies using dog models showed no direct influence on cardiac contractility, the increases in left ventricular dp/dt_{max}, and the cardiac output following pancuronium being dependent on heart rate.

As a consequence of a 25% average increase in heart rate, Kelman and Kennedy noted a mean 8.6% increase in cardiac output in patients under nitrous oxide phenoperidine anesthesia (41). The control heart rate in this series of 10 patients averaged 57 beats/min. A similar change in hemodynamics with less percentage increases in heart rate was recorded by Stoelting in patients under halothane anesthesia (30).

D. Gallamine

Gallamine also has an atropinelike effect which is limited to the cardiac muscarinic receptors (8). Experimentally, both vagal-induced bradycardia and bradycardia secondary to acetylcholine or methacholine are blocked. Gallamine has also been shown to release catecholamines from adrenergic nerve endings within the heart (21).

In man, gallamine produces increases in heart rate, principally by blocking vagal muscarinic receptors in the sinus node of the heart. This drug may have indirect sympathomimetic effects, but this action is probably less important than the vagolytic effect.

The tachycardia caused by gallamine has been shown to be dose dependent, reaching a maximum at approximately 1 mg/kg

(43,44). Nearly 100% increases in heart rate may occur if the patient's baseline rate is slow to begin with (in the range of 50-60 beats/min). Gallamine probably does not produce complete vagal blockade at this dose or at higher doses, since atropine given after maximum gallamine-induced tachycardia has been attained will result in a further smaller increase in heart rate (43). Gallamine-induced tachycardia generally persists beyond the neuromuscular-blocking action, such that heart rate slowing when gallamine is being used for operative relaxation may be used as a reliable indicator of diminishing neuromuscular blockade (45).

A rise in arterial pressure of 10-20 mmHg following administration of gallamine (44) is common, particularly under nitrous oxide narcotic anesthesia in the absence of potent anesthetic vapors. Increased heart rate secondary to the vagolytic effects of this drug in the absence of any fall in peripheral resistance is the probable mechanism involved.

Gallamine has been shown to have a weak positive inotropic effect on cardiac muscle (21,45). The mechanism may be increased catecholamine release within the heart or a relative shift of autonomic tone to the adrenergic side of the heart (21) owing to cardiac muscarinic receptor block. Some workers have shown a weak but not statistically significant positive inotropic action of gallamine in man (45). However, others were unable to show any positive inotropic effect in previously atropinized patients (46).

Tachycardia without any important change in peripheral resistance leads to an increase in cardiac output when gallamine is given to normal humans. Cardiac output increases are in the range of 25-50% after 0.5-2 mg/kg is given as a bolus intravenously. These are sustained for 5-20 min, and tend to be greater under nitrous oxide narcotic anesthesia than under halothane. Release of catecholamines in the heart by gallamine may contribute slightly to its effect on cardiac output (21).

E. Alcuronium

Alcuronium has a weak ganglion-blocking action and a relatively weak vagolytic effect at muscarinic receptors (11,47). This weak vagolytic effect of the drug may produce slight increases in heart rate, most notably when the baseline heart rate is slow (11,48).

Kennedy and Kelman (49), e.g., found a 9% increase in heart rate after 0.15 mg/kg of alcuronium was given to patients under nitrous oxide–phenoperidine anesthesia.

Although alcuronium does not release histamine (48) and only has a weak ganglion-blocking action (11,47,48), this agent has more or less been indicated as a cause of hypotension when large doses (0.2–0.3 mg/kg) are given to man (50–52), more notably in relatively ill patients (51). The hypotensive effect may be due to the ganglion-blocking action, since histamine release by alcuronium has been reported only once (53). Other studies have found that alcuronium has little effect on arterial pressure (49).

F. Vecuronium

Since the early studies on the pancuronium series the importance of cardiovascular side effects among neuromuscular-blocking agents have become apparent. Vecuronium was selected for study from a series of analogs on the grounds that it was the compound most likely to be capable of producing neuromuscular blockade without concomitant side effects.

Results obtained in anesthetized cats and dogs (Fig. 6) have demonstrated that vecuronium even in doses 20 times greater than those required for neuromuscular blockade has no effect on heart rate, arterial pressure, autonomic ganglia, alpha or beta adrenoreceptors or baroreceptor reflex activity (54,55). Studies in pithed rats and in guinea pig atria have also shown that vecuronium has little effect on cardiac muscarinic receptors or on norepinephrine reuptake mechanisms (54).

Eighteen adult patients under nitrous oxide narcotic anesthesia demonstrated no significant change in heart rate or arterial pressure with doses of vecuronium up to 150 μg/kg, which is three times the 95% blocking dose (56).

Equipotent doses of pancuronium and vecuronium were compared in 20 patients receiving halothane anesthesia. Pancuronium, 0.08 mg/kg, caused a significant increase in heart rate, an insignificant change in arterial pressure, and significant changes in systolic time intervals. The equipotent dose of vecuronium, 0.05 mg/kg, caused no significant changes in heart rate, arterial pressure, or systolic time interval (57).

G. Atracurium

Dose-response curves for atracurium obtained from results in anesthetized cats, dogs, and rhesus monkeys (Fig. 6) demonstrate that there is a wide separation between the doses required for neuromuscular paralysis and those that inhibit autonomic mechanisms (55,58).

In cats, significant hypotension and slight bradycardia were evident after administration of atracurium, 4 mg/kg intravenously, but this dose was 16 times that required for full neuromuscular paralysis. Similar results were found in rhesus monkeys.

In dogs, atracurium, 2 mg/kg, reduced mean arterial pressure to 53% of the control value, but this dose was eight times that required for full neuromuscular paralysis. Atracurium at high concentrations had no intropic or chronotropic effect on spontaneously beating guinea pig atria.

In man anesthetized with nitrous oxide and enflurane, there was no significant change in heart rate, mean arterial pressure, right atrial pressure, or cardiac output following administration of 0.2 or 0.4 mg/kg of atracurium (59).

In man under nitrous oxide narcotic anesthesia, mean arterial pressure and heart rate first showed significant changes from control values at 0.6 mg/kg, double the full paralyzing dose (60). Maximum heart rate and arterial pressure changes occurred 1–2 min after drug injection and returned to normal within approximately 5 min. These changes have been shown to be due to a dose-dependent release of histamine, and the increase in plasma histamine levels correlates with the heart rate and arterial pressure changes.

H. Succinylcholine

Succinylcholine stimulates both autonomic ganglia and muscarinic receptors, mimicking the action of acetylcholine at these sites (6).

The most common change in heart rate after the administration of succinylcholine is an increase (61–63), most notably in adults given small doses of atropine as premedication. The mechanism here is stimulation of autonomic ganglia, manifested as tachycardia because the vagal effect of ganglionic stimulation, bradycardia, is prevented by atropine.

The effect of a standard dose of 50 mg of succinylcholine on the circulation of human subjects premedicated with morphine, scopolamine, and atropine under nitrous oxide barbiturate anesthesia has been studied by Graf and associates (64). Under these conditions, resting heart rates were in the high normal range (mean 92/min) and arterial pressures averaged 107/79 mmHg; no further operative or anesthetic interventions were performed. In this series, a slight rise in arterial pressure (mean value after 3–5 min, 112/85 mmHg) was observed. The rise in diastolic pressure was more significant, being 7% above the control.

Repetitive 50-mg bolus doses of succinylcholine cause bradycardia in some subjects after the second dose; heart rate and arterial pressure changes after a third and subsequent doses demonstrated tachyphylaxis. Many other authors have also reported increased arterial pressure secondary to succinylcholine administration, particularly during prolonged infusion for maintenance and relaxation (6). Increased arterial pressure after succinylcholine administration may represent a clinical manifestation of its ganglion-stimulating action (Fig. 7).

Stoelting and Peterson (65) studied the hemodynamic changes produced by succinylcholine in combination with the circulatory effects of endotracheal intubation. Patients free of cardiovascular disease were given morphine and atropine as premedication and subsequently an induction sequence of d-tubocurine, 3 mg, pretreatment followed 3 min later by thiamylal, 4 mg/kg, and succinylcholine, 2 mg/kg. Larngoscopy and intubation of the trachea began 1 min after thiamylal and succinylcholine administration. Three minutes after the administration of thiamylal and approximately 2 min after intubation, a 5–10% mean rise in cardiac index above the preinduction value resulted in systemic vascular resistance increases of 10–20%, an increased myocardial workload being inferred. The cardiovascular changes were slightly attenuated by lidocaine (2 mg/kg) sprayed into the trachea before intubation.

In a group of patients (66) with coronary disease treated similarly, the cardiac index fell 10–20% in the face of a 25–35% rise in systemic vascular resistance. The hemodynamic data in this study when contrasted with results obtained in normal subjects infer a less effective myocardial response to the autonomic stimulus of intubation under the conditions listed above with

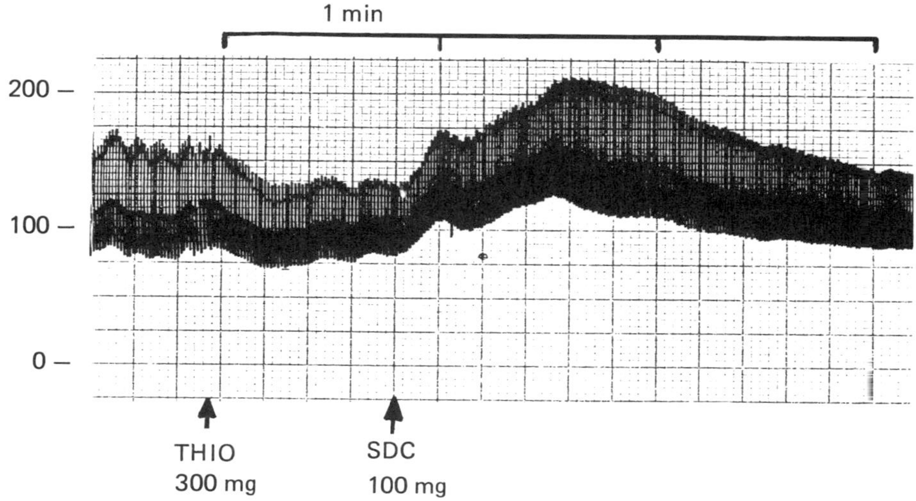

Figure 7 Hypertensive response to succinylcholine (SDC). Increased arterial pressure after succinylcholine administration may represent a clinical manifestation of its ganglion-stimulating action. This patient had a hypertensive response to succinylcholine. There was no other anesthetic intervention.

coronary artery disease. The data suggest that the induction sequence used is less safe in these patients than in normal subjects.

For the sake of comparison, it is worth mentioning that a similar study was conducted in normal subjects who were intubated under pancuronium- or d-tubocurarine-induced relaxation, at doses of 0.1 and 0.5 mg/kg, respectively, with a similar induction sequence (67). A 5-10% rise in cardiac index above preinduction levels occurred 2 min after intubation in the patients who had received pancuronium, whereas the cardiac index had fallen 15-20% after the same period in subjects who had received d-tubocurarine.

VIII. EFFECTS ON CARDIAC RHYTHM

A. Nondepolarizing Agents

The nondepolarizing agents generally do not in themselves produce cardiac arrhythmias. In fact, there is evidence that d-tubocurarine increases the dose threshold for the production of epinephrine-induced arrhythmias in dogs under halothane (68) and nitrous oxide anesthesia (69).

Arrhythmias after administration of pancuronium and gallamine may occur as a result of (1) a sudden shift of autonomic balance toward the adrenergic side owing to the vagal blocking effect of these drugs (2), a possible indirect sympathomimetic effect, and (3) a relatively greater inhibition of the atrioventricular node than the sinus node.

These mechanisms may manifest themselves clinically as single or multifocal premature ventricular contractions, ventricular tachycardia, or nodal (junctional) tachycardia. In the case of gallamine, junctional tachycardia may arise in patients with sinus node disease, the vagolytic effect causing a relatively greater increase in the spontaneous rate of activity of the atrioventricular node than the sinus node.

B. Succinylcholine

Succinylcholine is probably the only neuromuscular-blocking agent that may in itself precipitate cardiac arrhythmias in man under anesthesia.

Succinylcholine stimulates all cholinergic autonomic receptors, nicotinic receptors in both sympathetic and parasympathetic ganglia, and muscarinic receptors in the sinus node of the heart. The development of cardiac arrhythmias is a clinical manifestation of this generalized autonomic stimulation. Sinus bradycardia, junctional rhythms, and ventricular arrhythmias, ranging from unifocal premature ventricular contractions to ventricular fibrillation in special circumstances, have all been well documented. However, many authors of clinical studies have noted these arrhythmias under various conditions in the presence of the intense autonomic stimulus of tracheal intubation, and it is not always entirely clear whether the cardiac irregularities are due to the action of succinylcholine alone or to the added presence of extraneous autonomic stimulation.

Sinus bradycardia occurs most commonly in nonatropinized relatively sympathotonic individuals, e.g., children (70), and is due to stimulation of cardiac muscarinic receptors in the sinus node. Sinus bradycardia has also been noted in adults, and appears more commonly after a second dose of the drug given approximately 5 min after the first (71). It has been suggested that the higher incidence of bradycardia after a second dose of succinylcholine may be due to the hydrolysis products of succinylcholine (succinylmonocholine and choline) sensitizing the heart (72). Thiopental, atropine, ganglion-blocking drugs, and nondepolarizing relaxants have all been used to prevent the bradycardia.

Nodal rhythms commonly occur as bradycardias and are probably due to the relatively greater stimulation of the sinus node than the atrioventricular node. The result being a suppression of the sinus mechanism and the emergence of the atrioventricular node as the pacemaker. The incidence of junctional rhythm is higher (71) after a second dose of succinylcholine, but is prevented by prior administration of d-tubocurarine (73).

Succinylcholine lowers the threshold of a ventricle to catecholamine-induced arrhythmias in the monkey (74) and the dog (68) under stable anesthetic conditions. Other autonomic stimuli such as endotracheal intubation, hypoxia, hypercarbia, and surgery are probably additive to the effect of succinylcholine and may provoke ectopic activity.

Ventricular escape beats may also occur after severe sinus and atrioventricular nodal slowing secondary to succinylcholine administration.

The depolarizing nature of succinylcholine encourages ventricular arrhythmias by releasing potassium from skeletal muscle (75). This will be discussed in more detail in Chapter 7.

IX. DRUG INTERACTIONS WITH CARDIOVASCULAR EFFECTS

Succinylcholine lowers the threshold of a ventricle to catecholamine-induced arrhythmias. To this must be added the possible influence of drugs such as digitalis, tricyclic antidepressants, monoamine oxidase inhibitors, catecholamines, and anesthetic drugs such as halothane and cyclopropane, all of which may lower the ventricular threshold to ectopic activity or increase the arrhythmogenic effect of the catecholamines.

The nondepolarizing agents may also produce cardiovascular effects upon interaction with other drugs. A study in dogs (76) has shown that simultaneous administration of pancuronium and imipramine causes a tachycardia in an additive manner. The 80-μg/kg dose of pancuronium produced premature ventricular contractions and ventricular tachycardia, which rapidly progressed to ventricular fibrillation in two of the 10 dogs given imipramine, 8 mg/kg day, and in four of the 10 dogs given 16 mg/kg day. The authors concluded that severe ventricular arrhythmias may occur as a result of administration of pancuronium in dogs anesthetized with halothane and receiving imipramine chronically. In another study (77), neither pancuronium nor d-tubocurarine affected the arrhythmogenic dose of epinephrine during halothane anesthesia in dogs. This finding indicates that the usual guidelines for the administration of epinephrine during halothane anesthesia are not affected by concomitant administration of these two nondepolarizing muscle relaxants. Gallamine and d-tubocurarine (68) may decrease the incidence of epinephrine-induced arrhythmias in contrast to succinylcholine, which may enhance epinephrine effects.

Occasionally, drug interactions may be advantagous. Combinations of pancuronium and metocurine not only potentiate neuromuscular blockade (78) but also minimize the heart rate change associated with pancuronium on its own. At twice the ED_{95}, the heart rate increased significantly more in the pancuronium group than in the pancuronium/metocurine combination group.

REFERENCES

1. Meldrum BS: The actions of snake venoms on nerve and muscle. The pharmacology of phospholipase A and of polypeptide toxins. *Pharmacol Rev 17*:451–456, 1965.
2. Guyton AC, Reeder RC: Quantitative studies on autonomic actions of curare. *J Pharmacol Exp Ther 98*:188, 1950.

3. Burstein, CL, Jackson A, Bishop HF, Rovenstine EA: Curare in the management of autonomic reflexes. *Anesthesiology* *11*:409, 1950.
4. McDowell SA, Clarke RSJ: A clinical comparison of pancuronium with d-tubocurarine. *Anesthesia* *24*:581, 1969.
5. Moss J, Philbin DM, Rosow CE, Basta SJ, Gelb C, Savarese JJ: Histamine release by neuromuscular blocking agents in man. *Klin Wochenschr* *60*:891–895, 1982.
6. Paton WDM: The effects of muscle relaxants other than muscle relaxation. *Anesthesiology* *20*:453, 1959.
7. Birdsall NJM, Hulme EC: Biochemical studies on the muscarinic acetylcholine receptor. *J Neurochem* *27*:7, 1976.
8. Riker, WF, Wescoe WC: The pharmacology of flaxedil with observations on certain analogs. *Ann NY Acad Sci* *54*:573, 1951.
9. Saxena PR, Benta IL: Mechanism of selective cardiac vagolytic action of pancuronium bromide. Specific blockade of cardiac muscarinic receptors. *Eur J Pharmacol* *11*:332, 1970.
10. Marshall IG: The ganglion blocking and vagolytic actions of three short-acting neuromuscular blocking agents in man. *J Pharm Pharmacol* *25*:530, 1973.
11. Hughes R, Chapple DJ: Effects of non-depolarizing neuromuscular blocking agents on peripheral autonomic mechanisms in cats. *Br J Anaesth* *48*:59, 1976.
12. Li CK, Mitchelson F: The effects of stercuronium on cardiac muscarinic receptors. *Eur J Pharmacol* *51*:251, 1978.
13. Hughes R, Chapple DJ: Cardiovascular and neuromuscular effects of dimethyltubocurarine in anaesthetized cats and rhesus monkeys. *Br J Anaesth* *48*:847, 1976.
14. Hughes R, Chappel DJ: The pharmacology of atracurium: A new competitive neuromuscular blocking agent. *Br J Anaesth* *53*:31, 1981.
15. Durant NW, Marshall IG, Savage DS, Nelson DJ, Sleigh T, Carlye IC: The neuromuscular and autonomic blocking activities of pancuronium, ORG NC 45, and other pancuronium analogues in the cat. *J Pharm Pharmacol* *31*:831, 1979.
16. Loffelholz K, Muscholl E: Inhibition by parasympathetic nerve stimulation of the release of adrenergic transmitter. *Naunyn Schmiedebergs Arch Pharmacol* *267*:181, 1970.

17. Vercruysse P, Bossuyt P, Hanegreefs G, Verbeuren TJ, Vanhoutte PM: Gallamine and pancuronium inhibit prejunctional and post-junctional muscarinic receptors in canine saphenous veins. *J Pharmacol Exp Ther 209*:225, 1979.
18. Greengard P, Kebabian JW: Role of cyclic AMP in synaptic transmission in the mammalian peripheral nervous system. *Fed Proc 33*:1059, 1974.
19. Gardier RW, Tsevdos EJ, Jackson DB, Delaunois AL: Distinct muscarinic mediation of suspected dopaminergic activity in sympathetic ganglia. *Fed Proc 37*:2422, 1978.
20. Marshall RJ: A new muscarinic agent: 1,4,5,6-Tetrahydro-5-phenoxy pyrimidine (AH 6405). *Br J Pharmacol 39*:191P, 1970.
21. Brown BR, Crout JR: The sympathomimetic effect of gallamine on the heart. *J Pharmacol Exp Ther 172*:266, 1970.
22. Marshall RJ, Ojewole JAO: Comparison of autonomic effects of some currently used neuromuscular blocking agents. *Br J Pharmacol 66*:77P, 1979.
23. Quintana A: Effect of pancuronium bromide on the adrenergic reactivity of the isolated rats vas deferens. *Eur J Pharmacol 46*:275, 1977.
24. Salt PJ, Barnes PK, Conway CM: Inhibition of neuronal uptake of noradrenalin in the isolated perfused rat heart by pancuronium and its homologues ORG 6368, ORG 7268 and ORG NC 45. *Br J Anaesth 52*:313, 1980.
25. Lee Son S, Waud BE: Effects of non-depolarizing neuromuscular blocking agents on the cardiac vagus nerve in the guinea pig. *Br J Anaesth 52*:981, 1980.
26. Danilov AF, Kvitko IJ, Laurentieva VV: Action of some bisquarternary derivatives of phthalic acids and related substances on neuromuscular transmissions. *Br J Pharmacol 44*: 765, 1972.
27. Paton WDM, Zaimis EJ: Methonium compounds. *Pharmacol Rev 4*:219, 1952.
28. Everett AJ, Cowe LA, Wilkonson S: Revision of the structures of (+) tubocurarine chloride and (+) chondrocurine. *Chem Commun* 1020-1021, 1970.
29. Savarese JJ: The autonomic margin of safety of metocurine and d-tubocurarine. Abstracts of Scientific Papers, ASA Annual Meeting, San Francisco, pp. 393–394, 1976.

30. Stoelting RK: The hemodynamic effects of pancuronium and d-tubocurarine in anaesthetized patients. *Anesthesiology 39*: 645, 1973.
31. Antonio RP et al.: Unpublished data, 1977.
32. Dowdy EG, Holland WC, Yamanaka I: Cardioactive properties of d-tubocurarine with and without preservatives. *Anesthesiology 34*:256, 1971.
33. Stoelting RK: Blood pressure responses to d-tubocurarine and its preservatives in anaesthetized patients. *Anesthesiology 35*:315, 1971.
34. Antonio RP, Philbin DM, Savarese JJ: Comparative hemodynamic effects of d-tubocurarine and metocurine in the dog. *Anesthesiology 51*:S281, 1979.
35. Savarese JJ, Ali HH, Antonio RP: The clinical pharmacology of metocurine: Dimethyltubocurarine revisited. *Anesthesiology 47*:277, 1977.
36. Hughes R, Ingram G, Payne JP: Studies on di-methyltubocurarine in anaesthetized man. *Br J Anaesth 48*:969, 1976.
37. Zaidan J, Philbin DM, Antonio RP: Haemodynamic effects of metocurine in patients with coronary artery disease receiving propanolol. *Anesth Analg 56*:255, 1977.
38. Stoelting RK: Hemodynamic effects of di-methyltubocurarine during nitrous oxide-halothane anesthesia. *Anesth Analg 53*:513, 1974.
39. Nana A, Cardan E, Domokos M: Blood catecholamine changes after pancuronium. *Acta Anaesthesiol Scand 17*:83, 1973.
40. Miller RD, Eger EI II, Stevens WC: Pancuronium-induced tachycardia in relation to alveolar halothane, dose of pancuronium and prior atropine. *Anesthesiology 42*:352, 1975.
41. Kelman GR, Kennedy BR: Cardiovascular effects of pancuronium in man. *Br J Anaesth 43*:335, 1968.
42. Demenech SJ, Garcia CR, Sasian RJM: Pancuronium bromide: An indirect sympathomimetic agent. *Br J Anaesth 48*:1143, 1976.
43. Eisele JH, Marta JA, Davis HS: Quantitative aspects of the chronotrophy and neuromuscular effects of gallamine in anaesthetized man. *Anesthesiology 35*:630, 1971.
44. Stoelting RK: Hemodynamic effects of gallamine during halothane-nitrous oxide anesthesia. *Anesthesiology 39*:645, 1973.

45. Longnecker DE, Stoelting RK, Morrow AG: Cardiac and peripheral vascular effects of gallamine in man. *Anesth Analg* *52*:931, 1973.
46. Reitan JA, Fraser AI, Eisele JH: Lack of cardiac inotropic effects of gallamine in anesthetized man. *Anesth Analg 52*: 974, 1973.
47. Waser PG, Harbeck P: Pharmakologie und klinishe anwendung des kurzdauernden muscelrelaxans diallyl-nor-toxifern. *Anaesthesist 11*:33, 1962.
48. Savarese JJ: The autonomic margin of safety of alcuronium and pancuronium. *Anesthesiology* (in press).
49. Kennedy BR, Kelman GR: Cardiovascular effects of alcuronium in man. *Br J Anaesth 42*:625, 1970.
50. Baraka A: A comparative study between diallyl nortoxiferine and tubocurarine. *Br J Anaesth 39*:624, 1967.
51. Harrison GA: The cardiovascular effects of some relaxant properties of four relaxants in patients about to undergo cardiac surgery. *Br J Anaesth 44*:485, 1972.
52. Hunter AR: Diallyl toxiferine. *Br J Anaesth 36*:466, 1964.
53. Chan CS, Yeung ML: Anaphylactic reaction to alcuronium. *Br J Anaesth 44*:103, 1972.
54. Marshall RJ, McGrath TC, Miller RD, Docherty JR, Lamar JC: Comparison of the cardiovascular actions of ORG NC45 with those produced by other non-depolarizing neuromuscular blocking agents in experimental animals. *Br J Anaesth 52*:21S, 1980.
55. Sutherland GA, Squire IB, Gibb AJ, Marshall IG: Neuromuscular blocking and autonomic effects of vecuronium and atracurium in the anaesthetized cat. *Br J Anesth 55*:1119–1126, 1983.
56. Crul JF, Booij, LHDJ: First clinical experiences with ORG NC45. *Br J Anaesth 52*:49S, 1980.
57. Engbaek J, Ording H, Sorensen B, Viby-Mogensen J: Cardiac effects of vecuronium and pancuronium during halothane anaesthesia. *Br J Anaesth 55*:501–505, 1983.
58. Hughes R, Chapple DJ: The pharmacology of atracurium, a new competitive neuromuscular blocking agent. *Br J Anaesth 53*:31, 1981.
59. Hilgenberg JC, Stoelting RK, Harris WA: Hemodynamic effects of atracurium during enflurane-nitrous oxide anesthesia. *Br J Anaesth 55*:81S, 1983.

60. Basta SJ, Savarese JJ, Ali HH, Ross DM, Moss J, Gionfriddo M: Histamine-releasing potency of atracurium, di-methyl-tubocurarine and tubocurarine. *Br J Anaesth 55*:105S, 1983.
61. Barreto RS: Effect of intravenously administered succinylcholine upon cardiac rate and rhythm. *Anesthesiology 21*: 401, 1960.
62. Lupprian KG, Churchill-Davidson HC: Effect of suxamethonium on cardiac rhythm. *Br Med J 2*:1774, 1960.
63. Perez HR: Cardiac arrhythmia after succinylcholine. *Anesth Analg 49*:33, 1970.
64. Graf K, Strom G, Wahlin A: Circulatory effects of succinylcholine in man. *Acta Anaesthesiol Scand* (Suppl) *14*:1, 1963.
65. Stoelting RK, Peterson C: Circulatory changes during anesthetic induction: Impact of d-tubocurarine pre-treatment, thiamylal, succinylcholine, laryngoscopy and tracheal lidocaine. *Anesth Analg 55*:77, 1976.
66. Stoelting RK, Peterson C: Circulatory changes in patients with coronary artery disease following thiamylal-succinylcholine with tracheal intubation. *Anesth Analg 55*:232, 1976.
67. Stoelting RK: Influence of pancuronium or d-tubocurarine on circulatory responses during thiamylal-N20-halothane anaesthesia. *Anesth Analg 55*:485, 1976.
68. Tucker WA, Munson ES: Effects of succinylcholine and d-tubocurarine on epinephrine-induced arrhythmias during halothane anesthesia in dogs. *Anesthesiology 42*:41, 1975.
69. Wong KC, Wyte SR, Martin WE: Anti-arrhythmic effects of skeletal muscle relaxants. *Anesthesiology 34*:458, 1971.
70. Leigh MD, McCoy DD, Belton KM: Bradycardia following intravenous administration of succinylcholine chloride to infants and children. *Anesthesiology 18*:698, 1957.
71. List WFM: Succinylcholine-induced cardiac arrhythmia. *Anesth Analg 50*:361, 1971.
72. Schoenstadt DA, Whitcher CE: Observation on the mechanism of succinylcholine-induced cardiac arrhythmia. *Anesthesiology 24*:358, 1963.
73. Mathias JA, Evans-Prosser CDG, Churchill-Davidson HC: The role of nondepolarizing drugs in the prevention of suxamethonium bradycardia. *Br J Anaesth 42*:609, 1970.

74. Galindo AHF, Davis TB: Succinylcholine and cardiac excitability. *Anesthesiology 23*:32, 1962.
75. Bali IM, Dundee JW, Daggart JR: The source of increased plasma potassium following succinylcholine. *Anesth Analg 54*:680, 1975.
76. Edwards RP, Miller RD, Roizen MF: Cardiac responses to imipramine and pancuronium during anesthesia with halothane or enflurane. *Anesthesiology 50*:421–425, 1979.
77. Schick LM, Chapin JC, Munson ES: Pancuronium, d-tubocurarine and epinephrine-induced arrhythmias during halothane anesthesia in dogs. *Anesthesiology 52*:207–209, 1980.
78. Lebowitz PW, Ramsey FM, Savarese JJ, Ali HH: Potentiation of neuromuscular blockade in man produced by combination of pancuronium and metocurine or pancuronium or pancuronium and d-tubocurarine. *Anesth Analg 46*:575, 1974.

2
Histamine Release by Muscle Relaxants

RALPH P. F. SCOTT*
Harvard Medical School, and Massachusetts General Hospital, Boston, Massachusetts

**Present affiliation*: Southampton General Hospital, Southampton, England

I. INTRODUCTION

Histamine is distributed throughout the human body and is present in potentially lethal quantities in organs that are particularly vulnerable to its action (e.g., the airways, blood vessels, and heart). Most of it is sequestered with heparin in small membrane-bound granules in mast cells (3–20 pg of histamine per cell). These cells are imbedded in the mucosal linings, skin, connective tissue, and the tissue of small blood vessels and the conducting bundles of the heart.

Histamine was one of the first vasoactive substances to be identified in the body. It is formed by the decarboxylation of the amino acid L-histidine, a reaction which is catalyzed in mammalian tissue by a pyridoxal-requiring enzyme, histidine-decarboxylase (Fig. 1).

In mammals, histamine is metabolized by two routes. One involves deamination in the presence of diamine oxidase; the other, the methylation of the imidazole ring in the presence of the enzyme, histamine N-methyltransferase.

The widespread distribution of histamine in the mast cell is observed only in terrestrial vertebrates, but whatever the benefit of this particular development in vertebrate evolution, the mast cell is of practical importance to the clinician because of its ability to degranulate in response to allergic reactions and to a wide variety of drugs.

II. ETIOLOGY OF HISTAMINE RELEASE

Anesthesiologists encounter both immunologically mediated reactions and chemically mediated reactions associated with the administration of muscle relaxants. The explosive release of histamine from tissue mast cells and blood basophils by an energy-dependent mechanism may be in response to immunological or chemical stimuli.

The immunological reactions may be divided into:

1. Type 1 hypersensitivity response
2. Classic complement-mediated reaction
3. Alternate pathway activation of complement component C_3.

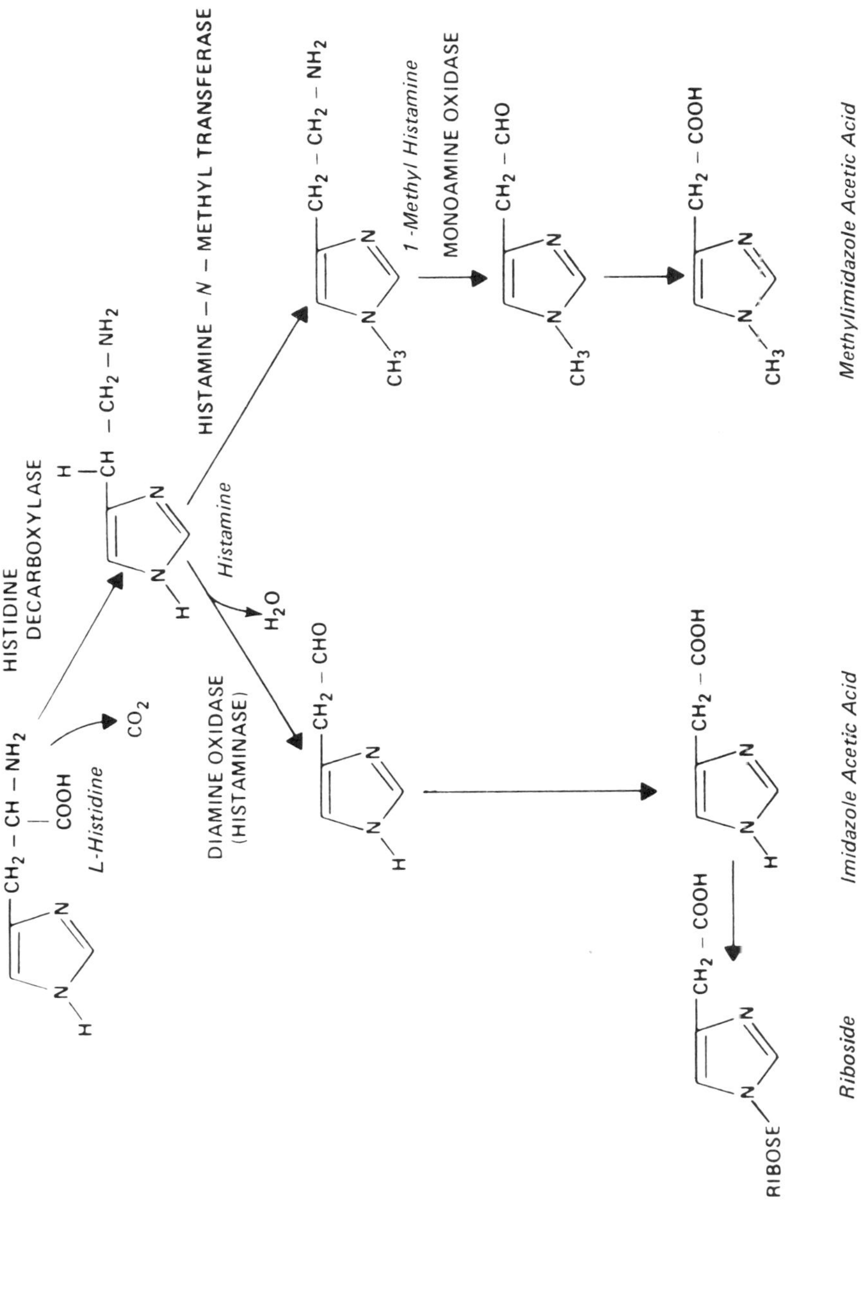

Figure 1 Histamine metabolism.

Immunological reactions to muscle relaxants have never attracted as much notice as those to intravenous induction agents. They are rarer but no less dangerous in their manifestations, since many may be severe enough to necessitate cardiopulmonary resuscitation. Reactions to succinylcholine are more common than with any other muscle relaxant.

Chemically mediated reactions happen much more frequently, and occur when the injected substance acts directly on the tissue mast cells and basophil leukocytes, leading to the release of histamine without antibody or complement involvement. Most organic bases may destruct mast cells and cause histamine release by this mechanism when sufficiently large doses or concentrations are used.

Several experimental studies have shown that histamine is released following the administration of certain neuromuscular-blocking agents, and that the histamine release is an important aspect in the hemodynamic response to the drug. This proposition is based partly upon preclinical and animal experiments in which various agents can elicit the release of histamine. However, the high dose of drugs required to effect histamine release in various in vitro studies as well as the species-specific characteristic of histamine release render extrapolation difficult. Thus, d-tubocurine can be demonstrated to cause histamine release from rat peritoneal mast cells (1), but the concentrations required to elicit this release is significantly higher than is achieved in clinical practice. The term species variability of drug-induced histamine release means that the animal models may not be a valid paradigm for histamine release in man. The rhesus monkey probably provides the closest parallel to the human situation, but even in this animal muscle relaxants tend to be more potent for the neuromuscular junction and less potent for histamine release, making the margin of safety for histamine release rather higher than in man. The margin of safety for histamine release by neuromuscular-blocking agents can be described for each drug. This indicates the number of multiples of the dose of relaxant producing 95% neuromuscular blockade that must be administered in order to produce the side effects associated with histamine release. That is,

$$\frac{\text{ED}_{50}\ \text{(histamine release}}{\text{ED}_{95}\ \text{(neuromuscular block)}}$$

In addition to the in vitro studies and animal experiments, there are a plethora of case reports (3) and clinical studies which demonstrate that the administration of neuromuscular-blocking drugs in usual doses can cause hemodynamic effects mimicked by the infusion of histamine (4).

III. HISTAMINE RELEASE BY MUSCLE RELAXANTS IN MAN

Most of the commonly used nondepolarizing muscle relaxants in the United States tend to fall into two groups. The steroids (pancuronium and vecuronium) and the benzylisoquinolinium compounds (d-tubocurarine, metocurine, and atracurium). Although histamine release by pancuronium has been described, it is classically a problem associated with the latter group.

In a study in healthy patients, Moss et al. (2) analyzed histamine levels with a radioenzymatic assay technique following administration of d-tubocurarine. While higher doses of d-tubocurarine caused increases in the mean levels of plasma histamine 2 min following administration, there was a significant variability between patients. It should be noted that mast cells from different species and even from individual tissues within a single animal are shown to vary markedly in their responses to given histamine inducers (5). However, it appears that there is a dose-response curve for d-tubocurarine-induced histamine release (i.e., as the dose of d-tubocurarine is increased there is an increased likelihood that the patient will release histamine). This ability to generate a dose-response relationship provides further evidence for a chemically mediated phenomenon rather than an immunologically mediated mechanism. Similar dose-response curves and similar variability for histamine release have been noted with other experimental benzylisoquinolinium neuromuscular-blocking agents, notably BW785 (6) and BWA444U (7). BW785 and BWA444U are interesting nondepolarizing compounds metabolized by plasma cholinesterase. BW785 has a significantly shorter duration of action than atracurium or vecuronium. Unfortunately, its margin of safety for histamine release was considered to be too low to be used safely. BWA444U had pharmacodynamic properties similar to that of atracurium, but again, its margin of safety for histamine release was considered to be too low.

The histamine liberated by muscle relaxants may produce a number of pharmacological effects dependent on plasma histamine levels. When plasma histamine levels are only marginally elevated (1000–1500 pg/ml) all that may be observed is a transient increase in blood pressure related to an increase in myocardial contractility. However, at higher levels (1500 pg/ml), histamine acts as a potent vasodilator. Thus, hypotension occurs, as does tachycardia, either as a reflex effect related to the hypotension or as a direct effect. Dilatation of cutaneous blood vessels with increased microvascular permeability results in flushing of the skin and increases in skin temperature. Stimulation of bronchial musculature results in bronchoconstriction. All of these effects are dependent on plasma histamine levels. Histamine also exerts effects on other organ systems, including the gastric mucosa, ileum, uterus, and the central and sympathetic nervous systems. The most frequent clinical signs observed by the anesthesiologist, however, are facial flushing, hypotension, and tachycardia. Therefore, the emphasis in this chapter will be on the hemodynamic effects of histamine release following the administration of muscle relaxants.

IV. HEMODYNAMIC EFFECTS OF HISTAMINE RELEASE

There is an abundant body of pharmacological literature on the effects of histamine in animals. More recently, a number of studies have investigated the effects of histamine on the human cardiovascular system. In vitro studies as well as a number of in vitro studies have demonstrated effects on the heart and systemic vasculature (8). Administration of histamine causes:

1. A chronotropic effect (H_2 directly and through catecholamine liberation)
2. An inotropic effect (H_1 negative, H_2 positive)
3. An effect on coronary vasoconstriction (H_1 constricts, H_2 dilates)
4. Changes in conductivity
5. Changes in fibrillation threshold (doses as low as 10 pg/ml)

In addition to the changes in the heart itself, there are important effects on the systemic vascular resistance which appears to be a direct effect of histamine (9). Recent studies have shown that histamine methyltransferase, one of the major catabolic enzymes for histamine, is located within arterioles, particularly in the kidney. The ability to maintain vascular integrity may depend upon the ability to metabolize endogenous histamine. It has been postulated that anesthetic drugs may interfere with histamine metabolism and thereby potentiate its effects.

Despite the significant variability in d-tubocurarine-induced histamine release, the increased levels of plasma histamine observed 2 min after d-tubocurarine administration correlates well with the observed hypotension (10). Multiple linear regression analysis demonstrates a tight correlation between the amount of drug administered and the amount of histamine released, and between the level of plasma histamine and the extent of hypotension (Fig. 2). The relationship between the dose of d-tubocurarine and the extent of hypotension is more tenuous. While d-tubocurarine has been shown to have ganglionic-blocking activity in animals, the contemporaneous restoration of hemodynamic variables and plasma histamine within 5 min of administration suggests that simultaneous ganglionic blockade is not involved and that histamine release is of more importance in terms of hemodynamic changes. Measurement of ganglionic blockade is difficult in the clinical setting, so that it is virtually impossible to establish how important a role it plays in normal anesthetized humans. Savarese (11), using the chloralose-anesthetized cat, established that ganglionic blockade induced by d-tubocurarine occurred at 1.31 mg/kg, whereas the delayed depressor response was transient and occurred at 0.4 mg/kg. Data accumulated during these experiments suggest that the duration of ganglionic blockade secondary to d-tubocurarine administration was similar to the duration of neuromuscular blockade. Classically, the histamine release observed with muscle relaxants is a transient phenomenon, with the associated hemodynamic changes returning to baseline within about 5 min. Histamine has a plasma half-life of less than 1 min.

Experiments with BWA444U (7), a muscle relaxant devoid of ganglionic-blocking activity, have also demonstrated a similar relationship between hypotension and plasma histamine 2 min following administration. It appears from these studies that the

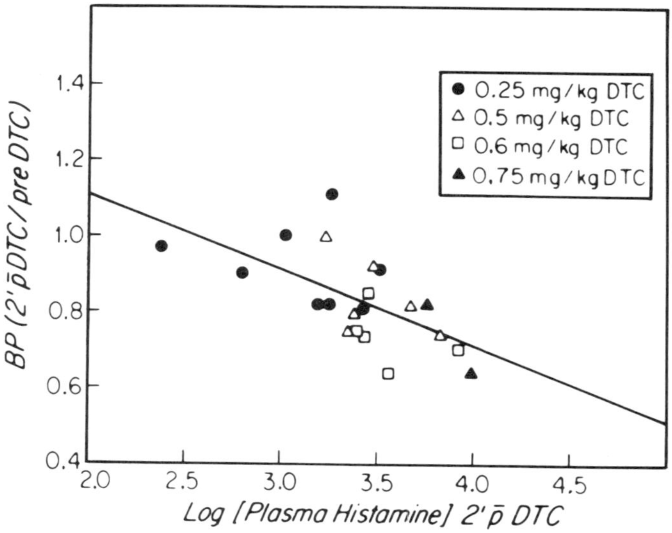

Figure 2 Relationship between the decrease in blood pressure and plasma histamine concentration 2 min after the administration of indicated doses of d-tubocurarine in 21 patients. (From Ref. 2, used with permission.)

dose of neuromuscular-blocking agent which increases plasma histamine to about 200% of control values will result in clinically and statistically significant changes in heart rate and arterial pressure in healthy patients.

Basta et al. (12) compared the histamine-releasing potency of atracurium to those of metocurine and d-tubocurarine. Atracurium produced a transient but significant reduction in mean arterial blood pressure at the upper end of its clinical dose range (0.6 mg/kg) (Fig. 3). However, when compared with other commonly used benzylisoquinolinium muscle relaxants, the ability of atracurium to release histamine relative to its neuromuscular-blocking potency was found to be approximately one-half that of metocurine and less than one-third that of d-tubocurarine (Table 1).

The other new intermediate-duration muscle relaxant, vecuronium, shows no histamine-releasing potential within the

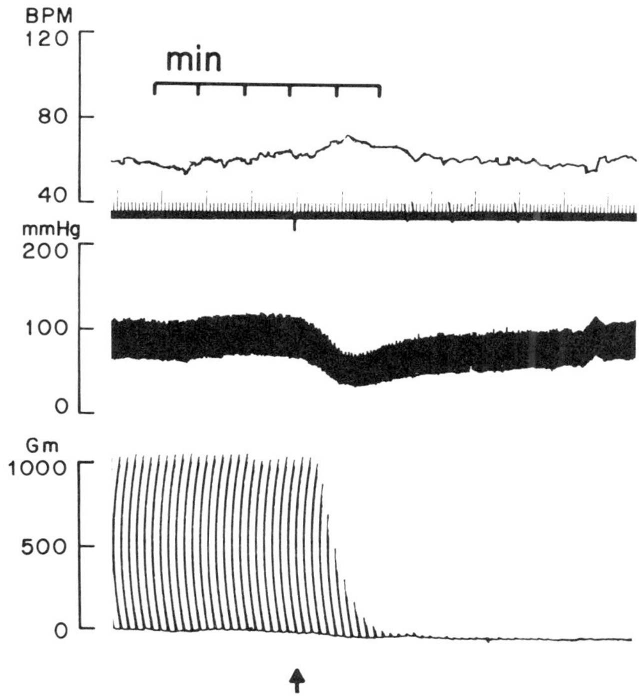

Figure 3 The transient hemodynamic response occasionally observed following a 0.6-mg/kg bolus of atracurium. Illustrated are the heart rate (by tachograph), intra-arterial blood pressure, and the single twitch at 0.15 Hz. Atracurium, 0.6 mg/kg, was injected as a rapid bolus at the arrow mark.

clinical dose range. Even at 0.2 mg/kg, three and one-half times its ED_{95}, there was no histamine release and hemodynamic parameters were stable. In a clinical study that measured skin redness and induration caused by the intradermal injection of d-tubocurarine, metocurine, pancuronium, and vecuronium, vecuronium caused the smallest reaction and d-tubocurarine and metocurine the largest (13).

Table 1 Histamine-Releasing Potencies of Neuromuscular-Blocking Agents

Drug	Dose (mg/kg)	$\times ED_{95}$	Percent of control		
			MAP	HR	Histamine
d-Tubocurarine	0.5	1	78	116	318
Metocurine	0.5	2	79	119	212
Atracurium	0.6	3	80	108	192
Vecuronium	0.2	3.5	99	102	87

Abbreviations: MAP, mean arterial pressure; HR, heart rate.
Doses of drugs associated with significant changes from control values. Note that even at $3.5 \times ED_{95}$, vecuronium has no significant change in cardiovascular parameters or plasma histamine levels.
Source: From Ref. 12, used with permission.

Succinylcholine has a histamine-liberating capacity of about 1% that of d-tubocurarine. Gallamine and pancuronium have minimal potential for histamine release within the clinical dose range.

V. STRATEGIES FOR THE ATTENUATION OF HISTAMINE-MEDIATED HEMODYNAMIC CHANGES

While the rapid administration of a neuromuscular-blocking drug can evoke hemodynamically significant histamine release, it has been shown that a variety of clinical strategies may be employed to attenuate the hemodynamic responses.

A. Injection Rate

In a study with d-tubocurarine, Rosow and colleagues found dose-related increases in plasma histamine occurring 2 min after injection in the groups receiving boluses but not in those receiving a slow infusion (Fig. 4). Even a 0.75-mg/kg dose of d-tubocurarine administered over 105 sec caused no clinically significant histamine release or hypotension (10).

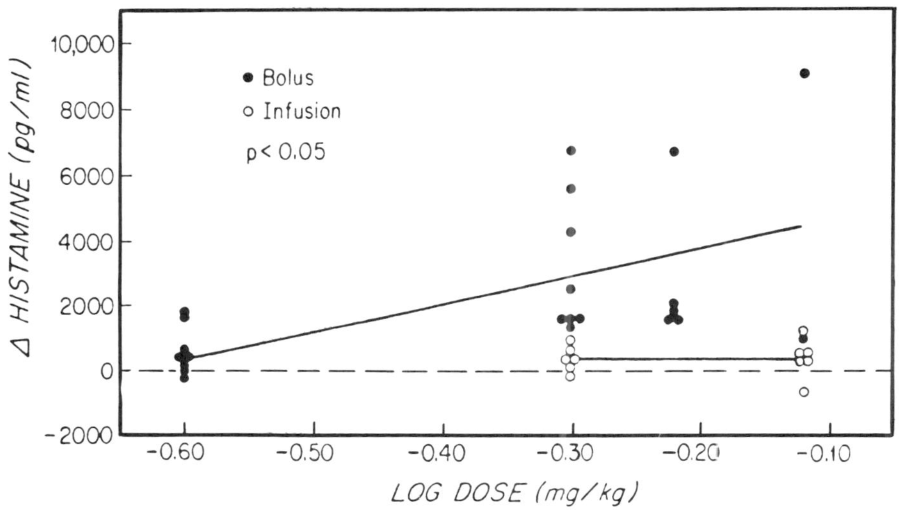

Figure 4 Slowing the injection rate of d-tubocurarine minimizes histamine release. In a study with d-tubocurarine, dose-related increases in plasma histamine occurring 2 min after injection in the groups receiving boluses but not in those receiving a slow infusion were found (10). (From Ref. 10, used with permission.)

In a similar study, a comparison of the alterations in hemodynamics and histamine release for BW785 following either a bolus or a 1-minute infusion of the drug demonstrated that when the drug was administered as a 1-min infusion it had significantly less hemodynamic effect than when administered as a bolus (6).

In a further study, the administration of BWA444U (1.2 mg/kg) as a 5-sec bolus caused significant increases in plasma histamine in several patients, whereas no detectable change was seen in any of the patients receiving the same dose in a 15- to 30-sec slow bolus (7).

More recently, it has been shown that the transient histamine release and associated hemodynamic response to high-dose atracurium (0.6 mg/kg) may also be prevented by administering this dose slowly over 75 sec (14) (Fig. 5).

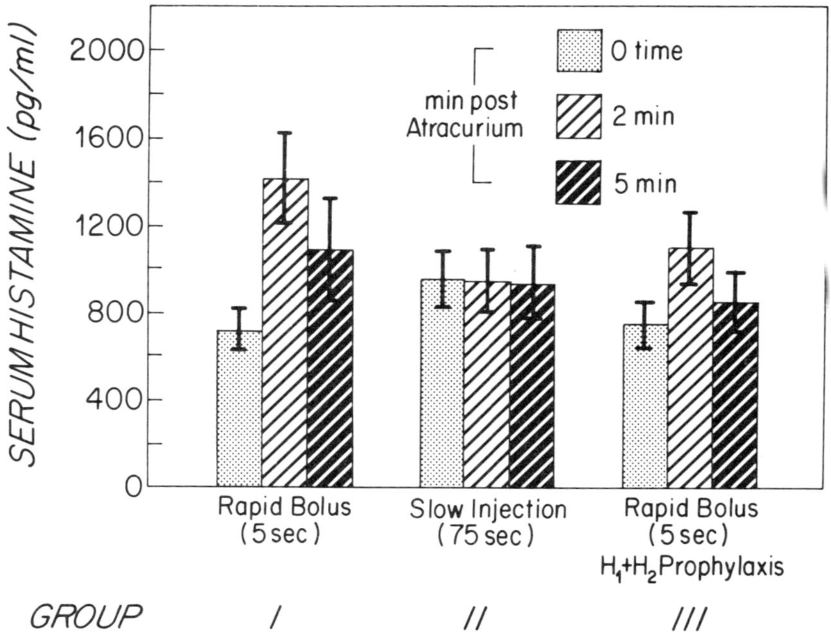

Figure 5 Histamine release by atracurium (0.6 mg/kg) and the subsequent hemodynamic response is prevented by administering this dose slowly over 75 sec. Pretreatment with intravenous H_1 and H_2 antagonists does not prevent histamine release but does attenuate the hemodynamic response. (From Ref. 14, used with permission.)

It thus appears that small time differences in the rate of administration of intravenous muscle relaxants can lead to significant changes in the likelihood of generating clinically significant histamine release. Small differences in plasma levels of a histamine-releasing drug can produce large changes in the amount of histamine liberated. Transiently high drug levels are more likely to degranulate mast cells.

B. Histamine Receptor Blockade

Aside from altering the rate of infusion, abundant data suggest that the prophylactic use of H_1 and H_2 antagonists can also attenuate the cardiovascular responses caused by various histamine-releasing drugs such as morphine (15), BW785 (6), haemaccel (16) and d-tubocurarine (10).

When cimetidine (4 mg/kg) and diphenhydramine (0.1 mg/kg) were administered intravenously 15 min prior to injection of a rapid bolus of BW785 significant cardiovascular protection could be achieved. It should be noted, however, that the rise in histamine levels following this approach was even higher than that seen following the injection of a single rapid bolus without anti-histamine pretreatment. This effect is presumably due to the known capacity of cimetidine to inhibit histamine N-methyl-transferase, which is possibly the principle route of histamine catabolism. Despite these high histamine levels, the cardiovascular effects were significantly less than in the nonpretreated subjects.

Similarly, when patients were pretreated intravenously with H_1 and H_2 antagonists prior to administration of atracurium, 0.6 mg/kg^{-1}, the hemodynamic response was attenuated (14), again despite a moderate rise in plasma histamine (Table 2) and (Fig. 5).

Table 2 Effect of 0.6 mg/kg^{-1} Atracurium on Mean Arterial Pressure and Heart Rate

	n	MAP % of Baseline	HR % of Baseline
Group I 5-sec bolus	9	82.1±6.4% (78.4/63.5/74.8)	108.5±4.6% (65/70.1/64.1)
Group II 75-sec bolus	9	95.7±2.6% (75.1/71.8/73.5)	97.7±2.3% (66/64.2/62.4)
Group III H_1 + H_2 prophylaxis before 5-sec bolus	9	96.2±2.2% (65.7/63.0/65.2)	102.3±2.2% (60.2/62.1/60.4)

Abbreviations: MAP, mean arterial pressure; HR, heart rate.
Actual values at baseline, 2 and 5 min for mean arterial pressure and heart rate are shown below in brackets. The units are mmHg and beats/min, respectively.
Source: From Ref. 14, used with permission.

The results of these studies using antihistamines are supported by pharmacological studies carried out in healthy subjects using systemic histamine (17). Exogenous histamine by rapid injection appears to stimulate only H_1 receptors. Chlorpheniramine alone antagonizes this response to histamine. The effects of cardiovascular H_2-receptor stimulation are demonstrated best by a sustained and a large dose of histamine given by infusion.

Experiments have been made in anesthetized cats and dogs and in healthy human volunteers to compare the changes in blood pressure and heart rate during the systemic administration of histamine (4).

Histamine (1×10^{-9} to 1×10^{-7} mmol/kg/min) lowered blood pressure in a similar dose-dependent fashion in all three species. In man and the cat, this was accompanied by a clear dose-dependent tachycardia, whereas in the dog, heart rate changes were minimal.

Pharmacological analysis of the depressor responses to histamine in all three species and the reduction in total peripheral resistance in the cat and dog showed that the immediate responses to histamine in all three species involved H_1 receptors, and that sustained responses involved H_2 receptors. Abolition of responses to histamine throughout infusions required H_1- and H_2-receptor blockade.

Therefore, in order to antagonize all the cardiovascular responses to endogenous histamine, pharmacological data suggest that this is best achieved by a combination of H_1- and H_2-receptor antagonists.

C. Drug Design

A third strategy in preventing histamine release involves structure activity relationships. Small variations in molecular design can radically alter the autonomic side effects of neuromuscular-blocking agents.

The histamine-releasing group of drugs includes a wide variety of different compounds. Indeed, the structures of these drugs are so diverse that Paton was forced to conclude that in addition to polymeric substances, any compound with two or more basic groups separated by a sufficient aromatic or aliphatic scaffold is liable to have this property. Even today, our knowledge of histamine-releasing structure activity relationships is still elementary.

The histamine-releasing properties of d-tubocurarine are probably due to the presence of the tertiary amine. In general, bisquarternary compounds do not possess strong ganglionic-blocking or histamine-releasing properties. Methylation of d-tubocurarine to produce metocurine or dimethyl tubocurarine (a bisquarternary compound) reduces the histamine-releasing and ganglion-blocking activities associated with d-tubocurarine.

VI. CONCLUSIONS

Since Alam et al. (1939) first detected the histamine release caused by curare, several thousand studies have been devoted to the question of whether or not histamine plays a significant role in adverse reactions to intravenous agents, and whether this role can be distinctly defined both qualitatively and quantitatively.

Unfortunately, the lack of a sensitive and reliable assay for plasma histamine had made it difficult to document the role of histamine release in drug-induced cardiovascular changes. The recent development, however, of a radioenzymatic technique and its improvement by the discovery of renal histamine N-methyltransferase has greatly enhanced our ability to detect histamine in clinically important situations.

The importance of histamine release in relation to the hemodynamic changes associated with the administration of d-tubocurarine and other benzylisoquinolinium compounds is now well recognized. One of the characteristics of an ideal muscle relaxant (18) is that this side effect be avoided.

Even atracurium has been criticized for its mild histamine-releasing effect when administered as a bolus at the high dose end of its spectrum. This side effect of atracurium must be kept in perspective. Atracurium has only one-third the histamine-releasing potential of d-tubocurarine, which has been used successfully for several decades. Also as outlined in this chapter, there are clinical strategies for preventing this response. In the health ASA (American Society of Anesthesiologists Classification) I or II patient, this transient hypotensive effect is probably of little clinical significance.

Nevertheless, in the hemodynamically unstable patient who is hypovolemic or has cardiovascular disease, this effect could well be of more importance.

There is no doubt that where a "clean" cardiovascular profile is required, vecuronium has to be the drug of choice. Certainly, with the new hemodynamic standards set by this drug, it is unlikely that the anesthesiologist will ever again see a new muscle relaxant introduced with a histamine-releasing potential greater than that of atracurium.

REFERENCES

1. Ellis HV, Johnson AR, Moran NC: Selective release of histamine from rat mast cells by several drugs. *J. Pharmacol Exp Ther 175*:627, 1970.
2. Moss J, Rosow CE, Savarese JJ, Philbin DM, Kniffen KJ: Role of histamine in the hypotensive action of d-tubocurarine in humans. *Anesthesiology 55*:19, 1981.
3. Lim H, Churchill-Davison HC: Adverse effects of neuromuscular blocking drugs, in, *Adverse Reactions of Anaesthetic Drugs* (Thorton JA, ed.), Elsevier, Amsterdam, 1981.
4. Owen DAA, Harvey CA, Boyce MJ: Effects of histamine on the circulatory system. *Klin Wochenschr 60*:972, 1982.
5. Pearce FL: Functional heterogeneity of mast cells from different species and tissues. *Klin Wochenschr 60*:954, 1982.
6. Rosow CE, Basta SJ, Savarese JJ, Ali HH, Kniffen KJ, Moss J: BW785U: Correlation of cardiovascular effects with increases in plasma histamine. *Anesthesiology 53*:S270, 1980.
7. Basta SJ, Moss J, Savarese JJ, Ali HH, Sunder N, Gionfriddo M, Lineberry CG: Cardiovascular effects of BWA444U: Correlation with plasma histamine levels. *Anesthesiology 50*: A198, 1981.
8. Bristow MR, Ginsberg R, Harrison DC: Histamine and the human heart: The other receptor system. *Am J Cardiol 49*: 249, 1982.
9. Rosow CE, Moss J, Philbin DM: Histamine release during morphine and fentanyl anesthesia. *Anesthesiology 56*:93, 1982.
10. Moss J, Philbin DM, Rosow CE, Basta SJ, Gelb C, Savarese JJ: Histamine release by neuromuscular blocking agents in man. *Klin Wochenschr 60*:891, 1982.

11. Savarese JJ: The autonomic margin of safety of metocurine and d-tubocurarine. ASA abstracts p. 393, 1976.
12. Basta SJ, Savarese JJ, Ali HH, Moss J, Gionfriddo M: Histamine releasing potencies of atracurium, dimethyltubocurarine and tubocurarine. *Br J Anaesth 55*:105S, 1983.
13. Booij LHDJ, Krieg N, Crul JF: Intradermal histamine releasing effect caused by Org-NC45. *Acta Anaesthesiol Scand 24*:393, 1980.
14. Scott RPF, Savarese JJ, Ali HH, Gargarian M, Basta SJ, Sunder N, Gionfriddo M, Batson AG: Atracurium: Clinical strategies for preventing histamine release and attenuating the hemodynamic response. *Br J Anaesth 57*:550, 1985.
15. Philbin DM, Moss J, Akins CW, Rosow CE, Kono K, Schneider RC, Verlee TR: The use of H_1 and H_2 histamine antagonists with morphine anesthesia: A double blind study. *Anesthesiology 55*:292, 1981.
16. Lorenz W, Doenicke A, Schoning B, Mamorski J, Weber D, Hunterlang E: Histamine release: H_1 and H_2 receptor antagonists for pre-medication in anesthesia and surgery: A critical view based on randomized clinical trials with haemaccel and various anti-allergic drugs. *Agents Actions 10*:114, 1980.
17. Boyce MJ: Pharmacological characterization of cardiovascular histamine receptors in man in vivo. *Klin Wochenschr 60*:978, 1980.
18. Savarese JJ, Kitz RJ: The quest for a short-acting nondepolarizing neuromuscular blocking agent. *Acta Anaesthesiol Scand 53*:43, 1973.

3
Muscle Relaxants in Patients with Neuromuscular Disorders

ISAAC AZAR
Beth Israel Medical Center, New York, New York

I. INTRODUCTION

Serious complications and even death may occur in patients with neuromuscular disorders following administration of muscle relaxants (1-20). Prolonged paralysis, hyperkalemia, rigidity, and malignant hyperthermia are the more common complications. This chapter reviews the response of patients with neuromuscular disorders to muscle relaxants, the possible mechanisms of abnormal responses, and the recommended management of relaxation during surgery. The malignant hyperthermia syndrome is discussed in Chapter 7.

I have classified the neuromuscular disorders according to the site of the primary lesion as follows:

1. Intracranial lesions: hemiplegia, Parkinson's disease, multiple sclerosis, diffuse intracranial disorders, tetanus
2. Spinal cord lesions: paraplegia, amyotrophic lateral sclerosis, poliomyelitis
3. Peripheral nerve lesions: peripheral neuropathies, muscular denervation
4. Neuromuscular junction lesions: myasthenia gravis, myasthenic syndrome
5. Muscular lesions: myotonias, muscular dystrophies

There are several methods to assess the response of patients with neuromuscular disorders to muscle relaxants. The regional curare test is considered the method of choice (21-23); the following is a detailed description of its administration and interpretation.

II. REGIONAL CURARE TEST

There are several different ways to perform the regional curare test, but they are all fundamentally similar. The following is the method used by Brown and Charlton (23): The patient's forearm is isolated from the general circulation by a tourniquet and curare, 0.5 mg in 20 ml of saline, is administered into one of the forearm veins. After 4.5 min, the tourniquet is released. At 1, 11, and 21 min after release of the tourniquet, nine supramaximal electrical stimuli at frequency of 3 Hz for a 3-sec period are administered to the ulnar nerve, and muscle action potentials of the abductor digitii minimi are recorded and analyzed.

If the fade of the train of muscle action potentials is greater and its recovery slower than normal, it is concluded that the tested subject has an increased response to nondepolarizing muscle relaxants. Conversely, if the fade is smaller and the recovery faster than normal, it is concluded that the tested subject is resistent to nondepolarizing muscle relaxants.

The fade in muscle action potentials can be expressed mathematically as the ratio between the first and the last muscle action potentials in a train. The greater the fade ratio, the greater the "sensitivity" of the patient to nondepolarizing muscle relaxants. The mean fade ratios in 22 normal subjects have been shown to be 1.76, 1.29, and 1.09 at 1, 11, and 21 min after the release of the tourniquet, respectively (24).

III. INTRACRANIAL LESIONS

A. Hemiplegia

Hemiplegia is caused by an upper motor neuron lesion in the cerebral motor cortex. It has been associated with resistance to nondepolarizing muscle relaxants (10,11,24) and hyperkalemia following succinylcholine administration (1,3,25).

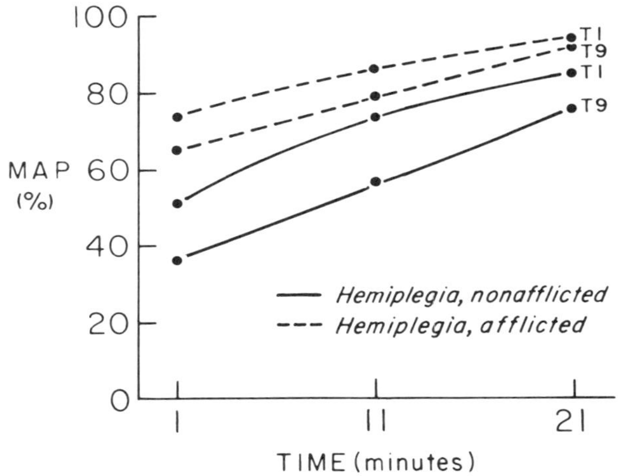

Figure 1 Mean train-of-nine values in 12 hemiplegic patients during recovery from the regional curare test. MAP (%), muscle action potential in percent of precurare values; T1, T9, the first and ninth responses, respectively. For more details see text. (From Ref. 24, used with permission.)

The regional curare test in 12 hemiplegic patients showed larger muscle action potentials and smaller fade ratios on the afflicted side when compared to the normal side (24) (Fig. 1). This suggests resistance to nondepolarizing muscle relaxants on the afflicted side. The degree of resistance did not correlate with the age or severity of the stroke. One patient with bilateral hemiplegia was resistant to curare on both sides. Two myasthenic patients who had sustained hemiplegia following cerebrovascular accidents had no clinical or electromyographic (EMG) signs of myasthenia gravis on the hemiplegic side (26).

Resistance to nondepolarizing muscle relaxants in hemiplegic patients also occurs during anesthesia (10). Following the administration of 9 mg of pancuronium in one patient, the "normal" side showed complete neuromuscular blockade, whereas the afflicted side showed no decrease in twitch response, no fade of tetanic response, and no posttetanic facilitation. In another patient, following the administration of 7 mg of pancuronium, the train-of-four ratio on the normal side was 0, and on the afflicted side 0.8.

It is not clear why the paralyzed muscles of hemiplegic patients are resistant to nondepolarizing muscle relaxants. Electromyographic studies of the paralyzed muscles show fibrillation potentials (27,28), slowing of nerve conduction (29,30), and reduction in number of motor units (31). Electronmicroscopic examination reveals loss of motor units and branching of the remaining axons (32). The new branches produce new neuromuscular junctions and extend the area that is responsive to acetylcholine beyond the neuromuscular junction. Eventually the entire muscle membrane is enveloped by receptors sensitive to acetylcholine. This phenomenon is common to all denervated muscles, and is called extrajunctional chemosensitivity.

It has been speculated that extrajunctional chemosensitivity is responsible for the resistance to nondepolarizing muscle relaxants in hemiplegic patients (11). This explanation is difficult to accept, since extrajunctional chemosensitivity also occurs in patients with lower motor neuron lesions (33), and yet increased sensitivity to nondepolarizing muscle relaxants rather than resistance is seen in the latter (5,6,34,35). Furthermore, the resistance to nondepolarizing muscle relaxants in hemiplegia is apparent as early as 2 days following a stroke, whereas the EMG and histological changes occur about 2 months later (31).

The early resistance to nondepolarizing muscle relaxants in hemiplegia suggests a possible central nervous system (CNS) effect at the neuromuscular junction. Brown and Charlton (24) speculate that normally there is an interplay between inhibitory and facilitative CNS effects at the neuromuscular junction and that in patients with CNS lesions the interplay is unbalanced. Depending on the level of the lesion, either facilitation or inhibition occurs. This would explain the opposite effects of cerebral versus spinal lesions.

Monitoring neuromuscular transmission on the afflicted side of a hemiplegic patient may lead to underestimation of the neuromuscular blockade and possibly to the administration of excessive doses of muscle relaxants. It may also lead to a premature discontinuation of ventilatory support.

Hyperkalemia and ventricular fibrillation following succinylcholine administration have been reported in hemiplegic patients

(1,3,25). Two episodes of cardiovascular collapse following succinylcholine administration occurred in a quadriplegic patient 1 week after a stroke (25). The serum potassium level during one of the episodes rose to 7.2 mEq/L. Succinylcholine-induced hyperkalemia was also reported in two hemiparetic patients (3). In one, 3 weeks following a stroke, succinylcholine caused a rise in the serum potassium level from 3.88 to 8.93 mEq/L.

The duration of vulnerability to succinylcholine in hemiplegic patients has not been established. Hyperkalemia may occur as early as 1 week (25) and as late as 6 months (1) following a stroke. There are no reports of hyperkalemia in patients with a stroke older than 6 months; still succinylcholine should be avoided if possible in all hemiplegic patients.

B. Parkinson's Disease

Parkinson's disease is an extrapyramidal disorder characterized by muscular weakness, rigidity, and tremor. There are no reports of abnormal response to nondepolarizing muscle relaxants in patients with this disorder. The regional curare test in eight patients showed a wide range of responses, but all were within normal limits (24).

There are conflicting reports on the response of patients with Parkinson's disease to succinylcholine. In one report (36), the changes in the serum potassium level were insignificant. In another (4), a rise in the level of serum potassium from 4.2 to 7.6 mEq/L and hyperkalemic electrocardiographic (EKG) changes occurred during succinylcholine infusion. The lack of other reports of hyperkalemia in this common disorder suggests low vulnerability and low incidence of succinylcholine-induced hyperkalemia in Parkinson's disease.

C. Multiple Sclerosis

Multiple sclerosis is a demyelinating disorder of the CNS, causing muscular weakness, numbness and parasthesias, visual disturbances, and occasionally myotonialike contracture of the muscles (37). The symptoms often get worse following anesthesia and surgery (38), probably owing to postoperative rise in body temperature (39,40).

There are no reports of abnormal response to nondepolarizing muscle relaxants in multiple sclerosis. In several reports, the response to alcuronium (38), curare (40,41), and gallamine (41) was normal. There is one report of hyperkalemia following succinylcholine administration (36). The lack of other reports suggests low vulnerability and low incidence of this complication in multiple sclerosis.

D. Diffuse Intracranial Lesions

Hyperkalemia and cardiac arrest have been reported in patients with diffuse intracranial lesions following the administration of succinylcholine (1,2,12,13,25). These patients had neither focal neurological deficits nor muscular denervation. In one report, the patient sustained two episodes of cardiac arrest 26 and 35 days after a head injury when succinylcholine was administered for tracheal intubation. The patient was successfully resuscitated and surgery was postponed on both occasions. A third attempt to anesthetize the patient without the use of succinylcholine was uneventful. In another report (12), a patient sustained two episodes of hyperkalemia and ventricular tachycardia 52 and 60 days after a head injury.

Potassium release following succinylcholine administration was also reported in a patient with terminal encephalitis (2). The serum potassium level rose to 10 mEq/L. Although it has been suggested that debilitated patients with disuse muscular atrophy may possibly sustain hyperkalemia following succinylcholine administration (42), this has never been reported in man.

Hyperkalemia following the use of succinylcholine has also been reported in patients with ruptured cerebral aneurysm (13,25). In a series of 22 patients, 10 to 50 days after the rupture, succinylcholine caused a 1–6-mEq/L rise in serum potassium in eight patients (13). Although some of the patients had motor paralysis, the degree of hyperkalemia did not correlate with the extent of the paralysis.

E. Tetanus

Tetanus is an acute infectious disease caused by *Clostridium tetani*. The bacteria release an endotoxin that blocks the normal inhibitory effect of the CNS on peripheral synapses and causes muscular spasticity and convulsions (43).

Nondepolarizing muscle relaxants were tolerated well by tetanus patients (44). The administration of succinylcholine caused hyperkalemia, up to 7.4 mEq/L, and cardiac arrest in two patients (44). Although it has been suggested that debilitated patients with disuse muscular atrophy may possibly sustain hyperkalemia following succinylcholine administration (42), this has never been reported in man.

IV. SPINAL CORD LESIONS

A. Paraplegia

Paraplegia is usually caused by a traumatic or pathological transection of the spinal cord and interruption of upper motor neuron tracts. Paraplegia patients show an increased response to nondepolarizing muscle relaxants (24) and hyperkalemia following succinylcholine administration (14,15,45–47).

The regional curare test in eight paraplegic patients showed an increased response to curare(24)(Fig. 2). This is in contrast to the response in hemiplegia, which is also an upper motor neuron disorder, where resistance to nondepolarizing muscle relaxants was observed (10,11,24). A possible explanation for this difference has been discussed earlier in this chapter in Section III.A.

The clinical implications of an increased response to nondepolarizing muscle relaxants in paraplegia depend on whether or not the respiratory muscles are involved: If the paralysis is limited to the extremities, the increased response to muscle relaxants is of little concern. However, if the respiratory muscles are involved, the administration of nondepolarizing muscle relaxants may cause postoperative respiratory failure. Continuous monitoring of the neuromuscular junction and reduced doses of muscle relaxants are recommended in these patients.

There are numerous reports of hyperkalemia and cardiac arrest following succinylcholine administration in paraplegic patients (14,15,45–47). The following was the sequence of events in one case (46): Immediately following succinylcholine administration, the patient developed bradycardia of 50–60 beats/min and

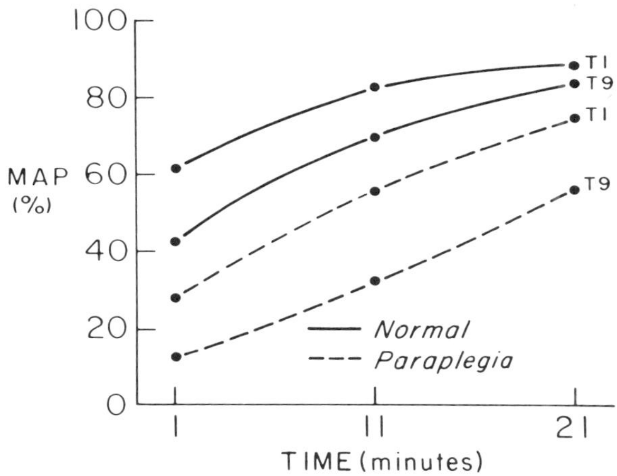

Figure 2 Mean train-of-nine values in 22 normal subjects and 8 paraplegic patients during recovery from the regional curare test. MAP (%), muscle action potential in percent of precurare values; T1, T9, the first and ninth responses, respectively. For more details see text. (From Ref. 24, used with permission.)

then tachycardia of 100–120 beats/min, followed by ventricular fibrillation. Cardiopulmonary resuscitation restored regular sinus rhythm within 3–4 min. Serum potassium levels measured at 5 min and at 3 hr later were 7.4 mEq/L and 3.4 mEq/L, respectively.

Tobey (47) observed cardiac arrest following the use of succinylcholine in four paraplegic patients 44 to 85 days after a spinal cord injury. He then studied another four paraplegic patients and determined the serum potassium level during succinylcholine infusion. Four minutes after the injection was started, hyperkalemic EKG changes were observed, and the potassium level rose significantly in all patients. Although the infusion was immediately discontinued, one patient sustained ventricular fibrillation. The blood potassium level returned to normal in all patients 5 min later. The blood potassium level in the inferior vena cava was significantly higher than in the superior vena cava. This suggests that the hyperkalemia is due to potassium released from the paralyzed muscles of the lower extremities.

The duration of vulnerability to succinylcholine in paraplegic patients has not been established. Hyperkalemia following succinylcholine administration occurred as early as 3 weeks (45) and as late as 85 days (47) after spinal cord injury.

B. Amyotrophic Lateral Sclerosis

Amyotrophic lateral sclerosis is a degenerative disorder of motor ganglia in the anterior horn of the spinal cord and of the spinal pyramidal tracts. The presenting symptoms are weakness and atrophy and occasional spasticity of the upper and lower extremities. There is a reduction in the number of motor units and an increase in the size of individual muscle action potentials (34). Histologically, sprouting of the remaining axons occurs (48).

Patients with amyotrophic lateral sclerosis exhibit progressive muscular weakness during exercise, fade of tetanic contractions (34,49), increased response to curare (24), and favorable response to anticholinesterases (34,49).

The cause of neuromuscular transmission failure in amyotrophic lateral sclerosis is not clear. One possibility is that the new motor end plates produced by sprouting axons in afflicted muscles are defective and "sensitive" to nondepolarizing muscle relaxants (35). Another more plausible explanation is that acetylcholine synthesis at the motor nerve terminals is compromised: The enzymes choline acetyltransferase and acetylcholinesterase, which are essential for the synthesis of acetylcholine, are normally manufactured by the anterior horn of the spinal cord and then delivered to the motor nerve endings along motor nerve axons (48,50). Mulder et al. (35) speculate that degeneration of the anterior horns in amyotrophic lateral sclerosis results in a reduction in the level of these enzymes at the motor nerve endings. This in turn reduces acetylcholine synthesis and causes neuromuscular junction transmission failure and increased response to nondepolarizing muscle relaxants.

The clinical implications of increased response to nondepolarizing muscle relaxants in amyotrophic lateral sclerosis are the same as those in paraplegia: If the paralysis is limited to the extremities, the increased response to muscle relaxants is of little concern. However, if the respiratory muscles are involved, the administration of nondepolarizing muscle relaxants may cause respiratory failure postoperatively. Continuous monitoring of the neuromuscular junction and reduced doses of muscle relaxants are recommended in these patients.

There are no reports of hyperkalemia following succinylcholine administration in amyotrophic lateral sclerosis. However, the muscular denervation and atrophy that often occurs in these patients is likely to be associated with potassium release and hyperkalemia. Succinylcholine should, therefore, be avoided in patients with significant muscular denervation.

A myotonialike contracture may occur following succinylcholine administration in amyotrophic lateral sclerosis patients (51). The characteristics and possible mechanisms of muscular contracture are discussed later in this chapter in Section V.B.

C. Poliomyelitis

Poliomyelitis is an infectious viral disease of motor ganglia in the anterior horns of the spinal cord and in the medulla. It causes flaccid paralysis of the extremities and may involve the respiratory muscles. Electromyographic studies of the afflicted muscles suggest neuromuscular junction dysfunction: The single muscle action potentials are small and tetanic responses fade (52–54). The cause of neuromuscular junction dysfunction in poliomyelitis is not known, but it could possibly be the same as that suggested for amyotrophic lateral sclerosis; namely, a decrease in acetylcholine synthesis at the motor nerve endings (35).

The clinical implications of increased response to nondepolarizing muscle relaxants in poliomyelitis are the same as in paraplegia and amyotrophic lateral sclerosis: If the paralysis is limited to the extremities, the increased response to muscle relaxants is of little concern. However, if the respiratory muscles are involved, the administration of nondepolarizing muscle relaxants may cause postoperative respiratory failure. Continuous monitoring of the neuromuscular junction and reduced doses of muscle relaxants are recommended in these patients.

V. PERIPHERAL NERVE LESIONS

A. Peripheral Neuropathies

Peripheral neuropathies are associated with systemic disorders such as diabetes mellitus, peripheral vascular disorders, metastatic neoplasms, alcoholism, vitamin deficiencies, and heavy metal poisoning (55). The clinical signs are sensory loss, parasthesias, and occasionally muscular weakness and atrophy. In some patients, the EMG resembles that of myasthenia gravis and suggests neuromuscular junction involvement, but these patients do not respond to anticholinesterases (56).

The regional curare test in patients with peripheral neuropathies is normal (24). However, resistance to succinylcholine (6) and increased response to nondepolarizing muscule relaxants (6,57,58) have been observed in patients with neurofibromatosis. Baraka (6) administered succinylcholine, 100 mg, to a patient with neurofibromatosis and observed no decrease in twitch response. He then administered 30 mg of curare and observed complete paralysis for 2.5 hr and partial paralysis for another 5 hr. In another patient, prolonged apnea was reported following pancuronium administration (58). The response of patients with neurofibromatosis to muscle relaxants resembles that of myasthenia gravis patients and suggests similar pathology at the neuromuscular junction.

An unusual response to curare has been reported in a patient with severe peripheral neuropathy associated with metastatic carcinoma of the uterus (59): Following 21 mg of curare, the twitch response decreased in a normal fashion, but the response to trains of tetanic stimuli remained sustained and no posttetanic potentiation was observed. The authors speculate that in severe peripheral neuropathies, the afflicted nerves fail to conduct the complete train of stimuli and that only a fraction of the original train reaches the neuromuscular junction. The decimated train is possibly too weak to cause tetanic fade and posttetanic potentiation.

There is one report of ventricular tachycardia following succinylcholine administration in four patients with long-standing polyneuropathy, possibly due to hyperkalemia (60).

B. Muscular Denervation

Muscular denervation is usually a result of traumatic peripheral nerve damage. The afflicted muscles undergo atrophy and the EMG shows fibrillation potentials (61). One to 2 weeks following the denervation, extrajunctional chemosensitivity develops and eventually the entire muscle membrane responds to acetylcholine (32).

The regional curare test in denervated muscles is normal, suggesting normal response to nondepolarizing muscle relaxants (24). The response to succinylcholine is abnormal and characterized by contracture (16,62–66) and hyperkalemia (62,67–69).

Muscular contracture is defined as an abnormal state of tension in a muscle, usually caused by an agonist such as acetylcholine or succinylcholine, and accompanied by total electrical silence. In contrast, muscular contraction is defined as normal state of tension in the muscle caused by an electrical stimulation and accompanied by muscle action potential (70). Muscular contracture may occur spontaneously or following succinylcholine administration in patients with denervated muscles (16,62–66), multiple sclerosis (37), amyotrophic lateral sclerosis (51), or myotonia (71).

There are several possible mechanisms for contracture: a prolonged and abnormally intense action of acetylcholine at the end-plate; an increase in the number of acetylcholine receptors at the end-plate; a decrease in cholinesterase activity at the end-plate (64); or extrajunctional chemosensitivity (16,33,62,63,65,72).

These theories are all based on the well-documented increased response of denervated muscles to acetylcholine (33): Smaller amounts of acetylcholine are required to produce muscular action potential and muscular contraction when compared to normally innervated muscles. These theories, however, are unacceptable because the normal response of the end-plate to acetylcholine is "all or none": Once the postjunctional membrane is depolarized, further potentiation of acetylcholine or succinylcholine would prolong depolarization and cause paralysis rather than muscular contracture. Also, the electrical silence observed during muscular contracture (33) does not support theories that are based on either increased acetylcholine receptor binding or repetitive membrane depolarization.

Jenkinson and Nicholls (73) showed that in chronically denervated and depolarized diaphragmatic muscles of rats, acetylcholine caused increase in ion movements across the membrane and produced a state of contracture without electrical activity. They also showed that the presence of calcium in the experimental bath was essential for the development of contracture. They concluded that in denervated muscles, acetylcholine promotes the entry of calcium ions into the cell, which in turn interact directly with the contractile elements inside the cell and cause contracture. This occurs independently of the contraction that normally occurs when acetylcholine binds with its receptors at the neuromuscular junction.

Hyperkalemia often occurs following succinylcholine administration in patients with denervated muscles. This has been well documented (62,67–69) and its mechanism reviewed (74). Twenty-two to 192 days after denervation, an average increase of 4 mEq/L was observed in blood samples drawn from the afflicted extremities (68). The blood drawn from normal extremities had significantly lower levels of potassium (67), suggesting that the hyperkalemia is due to release of potassium from denervated muscles.

A small dose of nondepolarizing muscle relaxants given prior to the administration of succinylcholine attenuates the ensuing contracture and the release of potassium in patients with denervated muscles (68). However, complete prevention of succinylcholine-induced hyperkalemia requires up to 0.5 mg/kg of curare (65). Pretreatment with nondepolarizing muscle relaxants, therefore, does not provide complete protection against succinylcholine-induced hyperkalemia. Succinylcholine should be avoided in patients with significant muscular denervation except during the period immediately following the injury.

VI. NEUROMUSCULAR JUNCTION LESIONS

A. Myasthenia Gravis

Myasthenia gravis is a disorder of the neuromuscular junction manifested by weakness and fatigability of voluntary muscles. Characteristics of myasthenia gravis are decremental response to tetanic stimulation, abnormally small miniature end-plate potentials, and reduced sensitivity of the end-plate to acetylcholine (75). Histologically, there are changes at the neuromuscular junction that suggest a decrease in acetylcholine receptor population (76). This was confirmed by using tagged bungarotoxins (77) and measuring miniature end-plate currents (78).

Most investigators agree that myasthenia gravis is a postsynaptic autoimmune disease that causes a reduction in the acetylcholine receptor population (79). Some still believe that a presynaptic lesion that interferes with acetylcholine production and release also exists (80). However, one report suggests that acetylcholine stores and acetylcholine release are two to five times greater than normal in myasthenia gravis (81).

Another possible cause of neuromuscular junction dysfunction in myasthenia gravis has been identified (82). Studies with sera of myasthenia gravis sheep suggest that antibodies in the sera occupy the ion channels of acetylcholine receptors and interfere with conformal changes that normally occur in the receptor subsequent to the binding of acetylcholine in the recognition sites. This inhibits ion exchange and renders the receptor nonfunctional.

The regional curare test in myasthenia gravis patients shows increased response to curare and prolongation of its effects (83) (Fig. 3). This suggests an increase in affinity between acetylcholine receptors and nondepolarizing muscle relaxants (84).

The response of myasthenia gravis patients to succinylcholine is also abnormal: Resistance and early appearance of phase II block have been reported (85-87). Many anesthesiologists, therefore, avoid muscle relaxants in myasthenia gravis patients and resort instead to volatile inhalation anesthesia for muscular relaxation (88-91).

The use of volatile anesthetics, however, also has drawbacks. Ether type agents, such as diethyl ether (88), methoxyflurane (92), and possibly enflurane and isoflurane, have a potent neuromuscular-blocking effect, particularly in myasthenia gravis. Low concentrations of diethyl ether or methoxyflurane cause muscular paralysis in myasthenia gravis patients, and because of their high partition coefficient and slow elimination, they linger in the circulation postoperatively and may cause postoperative respiratory failure. Also, myasthenia gravis patients with cardiac disorders may not tolerate volatile inhalation anesthesia. In such patients, the use of muscle relaxants should be considered.

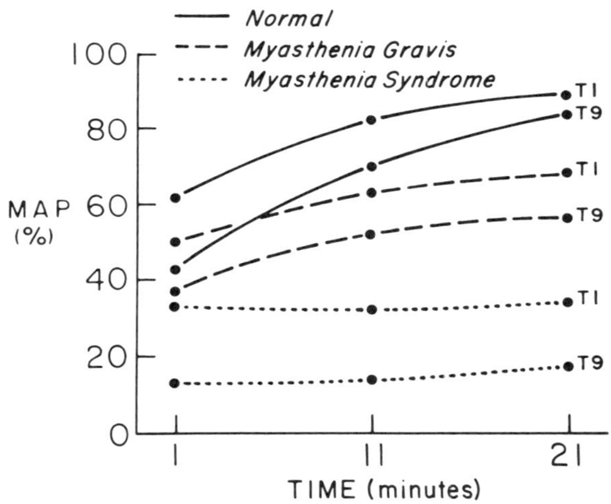

Figure 3 Mean train-of-nine values in 22 normal subjects, 21 myasthenia gravis patients, and two myasthenic syndrome patients during recovery from the regional curare test. MAP (%), muscle action potentials in percent of precurare values; T1, T9 and first and ninth responses, respectively. For more details see text. (From Ref. 24, used with permission.)

There are several reports of the uneventful administration of relaxants in myasthenia gravis patients. Baraka et al. (87) observed a normal response to succinylcholine. I observed normal relaxation and recovery following 1 mg/kg of succinylcholine given for tracheal intubation; however, the response to nerve stimulation suggested the early appearance of phase II block. Although recovery from a single dose of succinylcholine was uneventful, the effect of larger or repeated doses is unknown.

Pancuronium (93) and curare (I. Azar, unpublished data) in small doses have been used in myasthenia gravis patients uneventfully. As little as 0.005 mg/kg of pancuronium or 1.5 mg of curare was sufficient to reduce the twitch response by 90%. The recovery from these small doses was uneventful and no respiratory support was required postoperatively.

There are conflicting reports on the response of myasthenia gravis patients in remission to nondepolarizing muscle relaxants. The regional curare test in one patient suggested no improvement (83). Lake (94) reported 90% depression following 6 mg of curare during enflurane (1.5%) anesthesia. Based on this observation, Lake concluded that patients in remission remain "hypersensitive" to nondepolarizing muscle relaxants. The author's conclusion notwithstanding, the response of this patient to curare was normal: Enflurane potentiates the neuromuscular blocking effect of nondepolarizing muscle relaxants and significantly reduces the dose required to produce surgical relaxation (95).

In another report (96), a myasthenia gravis patient in remission had a normal response to curare: The patient was given 24 mg of curare during enflurane anesthesia and 45 min later the neuromuscular blockade was reversed promptly with neostigmine.

Despite the conflicting reports, it seems that myasthenia gravis patients in remission respond normally to nondepolarizing muscle relaxants. However, since remission is often incomplete, muscle relaxants should be used in small doses and the neuromuscular junction should be monitored continuously.

Special precautions should be taken in myasthenia gravis patients to avoid interaction of muscle relaxants and other drugs at the neuromuscular junction. Profound paralysis occurred in one patient who had recovered uneventfully from 1 mg of pancuronium and was then given thiophosphoramide (Thio-Thepa) and gentamicin (97). The latter two drugs potentiate muscle relaxants, and in myasthenia gravis they may cause complete paralysis. Similarly, antiarrhythmic drugs such as quinidine (98,99) and procainamide (99,100) should be used cautiously because they may aggravate the symptoms of myasthenia gravis and possibly potentiate the effect of muscle relaxants.

If possible, anticholinesterases should be discontinued the night before surgery, since they may complicate the anesthetic management. Anticholinesterases have a dual effect at the neuromuscular junction, and on occasion they may aggravate rather than ameliorate the symptoms of myasthenia gravis (101). In the presence of anticholinesterases, the differential diagnosis and treatment of postoperative respiratory failure becomes complicated. Also, if muscle relaxants are given during surgery, the anticholinesterases might prolong the effect of succinylcholine and antagonize the effect of nondepolarizing muscle relaxants. Some recommend discontinuing anticholinesterase therapy 24 hr prior to surgery (102) and others 1-4 days earlier (90).

B. Myasthenic Syndrome

Myasthenic syndrome differs clinically and electromyographically from myasthenia gravis. It occurs mostly in males 50-70 years old and is associated with small cell carcinoma of the lung (103,104) and other malignancies (105). The symptoms are fatigability and aches in the proximal muscles of the extremities. Unlike myasthenia gravis patients, myasthenic syndrome patients experience an increase in muscle strength with exercise, they respond poorly to anticholinesterases, and they have an exaggerated response to depolarizing and nondepolarizing muscle relaxants (8).

The pathology of myasthenic syndrome is at the motor nerve ending of the neuromuscular junction (26,81). Although the number and contents of the acetylcholine vesicles are normal, the release of acetylcholine is slower than normal (81,106).

The response of myasthenic syndrome patients to curare is greater than in myasthenia gravis patients (83). The regional curare test in two myasthenic syndrome patients was compared to that of myasthenia gravis patients and it showed smaller muscle action potentials and greater fade ratios in the myasthenic syndrome patients (Fig. 3). In one case report, 5 mg of curare caused paralysis that lasted 24 hr (8).

VII. MUSCULAR LESIONS

A. Myotonias

The myotonias are characterized by a delayed relaxation of skeletal muscles following voluntary contractions. The lesion is in the muscle fiber proper distal to the neuromuscular junction, but its exact nature is uncertain (107-110). Repetitive nerve stimulation causes a gradual and sustained increase in muscle tension without concomitant muscle action potentials (111).

Sprouting of motor nerve axons, extrajunctional chemosensitivity (112), and a decrease in the cholinesterase level at the neuromuscular junction (110) have been observed in afflicted muscles.

There are conflicting reports on the response of myotonic patients to nondepolarizing muscle relaxants. The regional curare test in 12 patients was normal (24). The response to "usual" clinical doses of curare (113-116) and pancuronium (117) was also normal. However, there is one case report of paralysis lasting 3.5 hr after administration of 25 mg of curare (118).

Since myotonias are often associated with dystrophic muscular changes, it is conceivable that in advanced cases there will be an increased response to nondepolarizing muscle relaxants. The dose of muscle relaxants should be reduced according to the extent of muscular waste, and the neuromuscular junction should be monitored continuously during surgery.

The response of myotonic patients to succinylcholine is unpredictable. Some report normal response (116,119-121), others generalized myotonia and ventilatory failure (7,17,122), and still others relaxation of muscles that are in a myotonic state (123,124). A test dose of 3 mg of succinylcholine given to two myotonic siblings had no effect on one, and caused generalized contracture and respiratory distress in the other (125).

Thiel (122) described a typical myotonic response to succinylcholine: One minute following the administration of succinylcholine, generalized spasm developed, the jaw became rigid, the abdomen tight, the limbs flexed, and the cervical and lumbar spine arched. Respiration ceased. Two minutes later, the jaw relaxed but intubation was impossible until 4 min later. The duration of the apnea following succinylcholine administration was within normal limits. The recovery of spontaneous breathing and the relaxation of the myotonic contracture occurred simultaneously.

A more severe response to succinylcholine, complicated by laryngospasm and cyanosis, was reported in a patient with myotonia congenita (7). The myotonic contracture resolved spontaneously and respiration returned to normal 3.5 min later.

In a prospective study of myotonic patients, all subjects developed dose-dependent generalized contracture following the administration of succinylcholine (51). A dose larger than 40 mg did not increase the intensity of the contracture, and multiple doses caused tachyphylaxis and a decrease in the myotonic state.

The mechanical response of myotonic muscles to succinylcholine suggests a dual effect of succinylcholine at the neuromuscular junction of these muscles (51,126): The twitch response decreases as usual, but at the same time tension develops in the muscle in a dose-dependent fashion (Fig. 4). This explains the simultaneous onset of respiratory depression and of muscular contracture following succinylcholine administration.

The similar contracture seen in myotonic and denervated muscles following succinylcholine suggests similar pathophysiology at the neuromuscular junction: abnormal ion channels (127) and abnormal entry of calcium ions into the muscle during depolarizing (73). The therapeutic effectiveness in myotonia of two well-known ion-channel blockers, quinidine and procainamide (128), supports this hypothesis. A complete discussion on muscular contracture can be found in Section V.B. in this chapter.

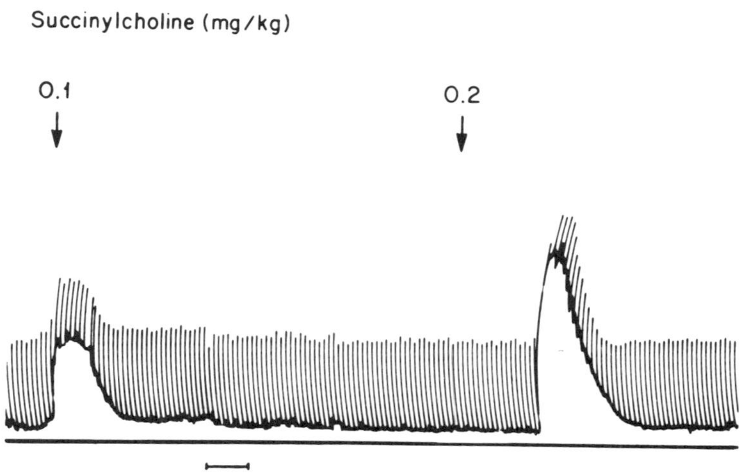

Figure 4 The response of a myotonic patient to succinylcholine. The depression in twitch response occurred concomitantly with an increase in baseline tension of the muscle. (From Ref. 126, used with permission.)

The rigidity induced by succinylcholine in myotonic patients is similar to that observed in patients with malignant hyperthermia syndrome. This suggests a possible association between the two disorders. There are indeed two case reports of malignant hyperthermia following succinylcholine in myotonic patients (18,129); however, muscle biopsies studied in five myotonic patients were negative for malignant hyperthermia (130). It is generally believed that there is no increase in susceptibility to malignant hyperthermia in myotonia (130–132).

Since the response of myotonic patients to succinylcholine is unpredictable, it is recommended that succinylcholine be avoided in these patients.

A major problem in the anesthetic management of myotonic patients is the lack of surgical relaxation owing to spontaneous onset of myotonic contracture during surgery. Since the pathology is located in the muscle fiber proper, neither muscle relaxants (108,133) nor regional anesthesia (107,110,134,135) alleviate the contracture. Only drugs with a direct effect on the muscle membrane such as quinine (51,124,136), procainamide (124,133, 137), local anesthetics (110,135,138), diphenylhydantoin (139), volatile anesthetic agents (117), and steroids (137) can attenuate the myotonic contracture.

Procainamide and prednisone are equally effective in attenuating myotonic contracture (137). Significant improvement was observed in two patients following 0.8–1 gm of procainamide, although "percussion" myotonia, triggered by the surgeon's handling of the muscles, remained unchanged (133). Potent inhalation anesthetics are usually effective, but at the cost of cardiovascular depression. "High" inspiratory concentration of halothane failed to relax myotonic contracture and did not facilitate tracheal intubation in one patient (125). Althesin, an intravenous anesthetic agent commonly used in Europe but not approved in the United States, has a direct muscle-relaxing effect and is recommended in the anesthetic management of myotonic patients (117).

When everything else fails, infiltration of the muscles around the surgical incision with a local anesthetic is recommended (110,135,137).

Potassium (134), neostigmine (134,140), and hypothermia and shivering (122) provoke myotonic contracture. Potassium administration should be avoided except in cases of life-threatening hypokalemia. Neostigmine should be avoided if possible, although it has been used without complications (110,116,126). Shivering may trigger myotonic contracture and should be avoided by placing the patient on a thermal blanket and raising the room temperature to a level comfortable to the patient.

B. Muscular Dystrophies

The muscular dystrophies are primarily disorders of the muscle fiber proper, although some believe that they are secondary to a neurogenic disorder (141-144). Pathological changes had been observed in the neuromuscular junction of muscular dystrophy patients (143) and mice (142) well before the dystrophic changes appeared in the muscle fiber proper.

There are conflicting reports on the response of muscular dystrophy patients to nondepolarizing muscle relaxants. The regional curare test in 11 patients showed a normal initial response to curare, but the block lasted significantly longer than normal (24) (Fig. 5). However, the response during surgery to gallamine (124,145) and curare (145) was reported as "normal."

One particular type of muscular dystrophy, the ocular type, exhibits exquisite "sensitivity" to curare, similar to that seen in myasthenia gravis. Unlike patients with myasthenia gravis, however, patients with ocular muscular dystrophy respond poorly to anticholinesterase therapy (19,146,147).

Different responses to succinylcholine have been reported in patients with muscular dystrophy. Normal response was reported in large series (122,145). In contrast, cardiac arrest was reported in four patients (20,145,148). The patients were resuscitated and they all recovered uneventfully except for postoperative myoglobinuria in one and elevated creatine phosphokinase (CPK) in another (20). Although serum potassium levels were not determined, hyperkalemia was suspected as the cause of cardiac arrest in these patients.

Serum levels of CPK and other intracellular enzymes are often elevated in patients with muscular dystrophy (145).

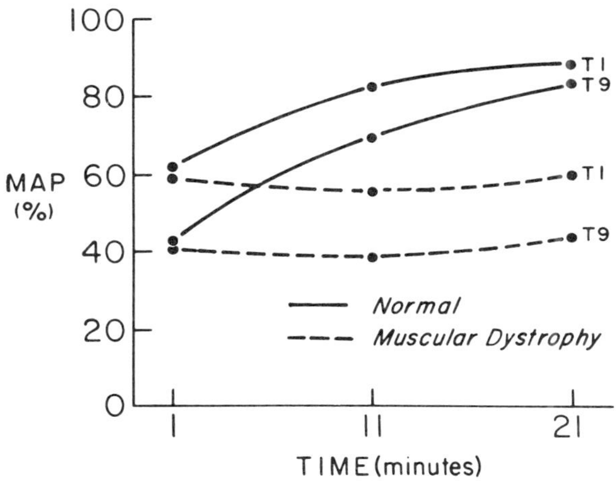

Figure 5 Mean train-of-nine values in 22 normal subjects and 11 muscular dystrophy patients during recovery from the regional curare test. MAP (%), muscle action potential in percent of precurare values. T1, T9, the first and the ninth responses, respectively. For more details see text. (From Ref. 24, used with permission.)

Although malignant hyperthermia has been associated with elevated serum CPK (149), this syndrome did not occur in a series of 43 muscular dystrophy patients who were operated upon under general anesthesia. However, there are several other reports of atypical malignant hyperthermia, and in some of these patients the muscle biopsy studies for malignant hyperthermia were positive (150-155). Based on these reports, it has been suggested that muscular dystrophy patients are more likely to sustain malignant hyperthermia than the general population (156); however, this has not been substantiated statistically.

Since the response of muscular dystrophy patients to succinylcholine is unpredictable, it is recommended that succinylcholine be avoided in these patients.

VIII. RIGIDITY FOLLOWING SUCCINYLCHOLINE ADMINISTRATION

Rigidity following succinylcholine administration, particularly that of the jaw, occurs occasionally (16,51,63-69,157-163). Although this may be a prelude to malignant hyperthermia (163), other disorders should also be considered. Rigidity has been reported in myotonia (17,51), muscular dystrophy (20), amyotrophic lateral sclerosis (51), chronically denervated muscles (16,63-66), polymyositis (18,147), and mitochondrial myopathies (161,162). Since the clinical symptoms of dystrophic myotonia are not apparent until the third decade of life (158), some of the unexplained cases of rigidity are probably due to undiagnosed myotonia. Occasionally, the cause for rigidity cannot be determined.

Rigidity has also been associated with a particular syndrome described as hypermetabolic muscular derangement (159). This particular syndrome shares several features with malignant hyperthermia: Following the administration of succinylcholine, the patient becomes rigid, the body temperature rises moderately (usually not higher than 38°C), and mild metabolic and respiratory acidosis develop. The patient recovers uneventfully except for postoperative myalgia and myoglobinuria. Muscle biopsy studies for malignant hyperthermia are negative (158,159).

The rigidity induced by succinylcholine in myotonic patients is usually self-limited and benign, whereas in malignant hyperthermia it may be a prelude to a catastrophe. It is important, therefore, to distinguish between the two as early as possible. One difference is the duration of the rigidity: In myotonia, the rigidity is short lived, lasting only as long as the normal paralyzing effect of succinylcholine; in malignant hyperthermia, the rigidity lingers well after the normal paralyzing effect of succinylcholine dissipates (158,163).

When a patient becomes rigid following succinylcholine administration, postponement of surgery should be considered, particularly if it is accompanied by a rise in heart rate, temperature, or blood carbon dioxide level. Cody (17) reviewed the literature and observed that when patients had developed rigidity following succinylcholine, three out of four died if surgery was continued and three out of four survived if surgery was postponed.

REFERENCES

1. Smith RB, Grenvik, A: Cardiac arrest following succinylcholine in patients with central nervous system injuries. *Anesthesiology 33*:558-560, 1970.
2. Cowgill DB, Mostello LA, Shapiro HM: Encephalitis and a hyperkalemic response to succinylcholine. *Anesthesiology 40*:409-411, 1974.
3. Cooperman LH, Strobel GE Jr, Kennell EM: Massive hyperkalemia after administration of succinylcholine. *Anesthesiology 32*:161-164, 1979.
4. Gravlee GP: Succinylcholine-induced hyperkalemia in a patient with Parkinson's disease. *Anesth Analg 59*:444-446, 1980.
5. Rosenbaum KJ, Neigh JL, Strobel GE: Sensitivity to non-depolarizing muscle relaxants in amyotrophic lateral sclerosis: Report of two cases. *Anesthesiology 35*:638-641, 1971.
6. Baraka A: Myasthenic response to muscle relaxants in Von Recklinghausen's disease. *Br J Anaesth 46*:701-703, 1974.
7. Paterson IS: Generalized myotonia following suxamethonium. *Br J Anaesth 34*:340-342, 1962.
8. Wise RP: A myasthenic syndrome complicating bronchial carcinoma. *Br J Anaesth 17*:488-504, 1962.
9. Colp C, Kriplani L, Nussbaum M: Vocal cords paralysis in myasthenia gravis following anesthesia. *Chest 77*:218-220, 1980.
10. Graham DH: Monitoring neuromuscular block may be unreliable in patients with upper-motor-neurone lesions. *Anesthesiology 52*:74-75, 1980.
11. Moorthy SS, Hilgenberg JC: Resistance to non-depolarizing muscle relaxants in paretic upper extremities of patients with residual hemiplegia. *Anesth Analg 59*:624-627, 1980.
12. Stevenson PH, Birch AA: Succinylcholine-induced hyperkalemia in a patient with a closed head injury. *Anesthesiology 51*:89-90, 1979.
13. Iwatsuki N, Kuroda N, Omaha K, Iwatsuki K: Succinylcholine-induced hyperkalemia in patients with ruptured cerebral aneurysm. *Anesthesiology 53*:64-67, 1980.
14. Snow JC, Kripke BJ, Sessions GP, Finck AJ: Cardiovascular collapse following succinylcholine in a paraplegic patient. *Paraplegia 11*:199-204, 1973.

15. Walker DE, Barry JM, Hodges CV: Succinylcholine-induced ventricular fibrillation in the paralyzed urology patient. *J. Urol 113*:111-113, 1975.
16. Baraka A: Suxamethonium-induced muscle contracture following traumatic denervation in man. *Br J Anaesth 50*: 195-199, 1978.
17. Cody JR: Muscle rigidity following administration of succinylcholine. *Anesthesiology 29*:159-162, 1968.
18. Saidman, LJ, Havard ES, Eger IE: Hyperthermia during anesthesia. *JAMA 190*:1029-1032, 1964.
19. Jacob, JC, Varkey GP: Curare sensitivity in ocular myopathy. *Can Anaesth Soc J 13*:449-452, 1966.
20. Seay AR, Ziter FA, Thompson JA: Cardiac arrest during induction of anesthesia in Duchenne muscular dystrophy. *J Pediatr 93*:88-90, 1978.
21. Foldes FF, Glaser GH: Diagnostic tests in myasthenia gravis: An overview. *Ann NY Acad Sci 183*:275-286, 1971.
22. Foldes FF, Klonymus DH, Maisel W, Osserman KE: A new curare test for the diagnosis of myasthenia gravis. *JAMA 203*:133-137, 1968.
23. Brown JC, Charlton JE, White DJK: A regional technique for the study of sensitivity to curare in human muscle. *J Neurol Neurosurg Psychiatr 38*:18-26, 1975.
24. Brown JC, Charlton JE: Study of sensitivity to curare in certain neurological disorders using a regional technique. *J Neurol Neurosurg Psychiatr 38*:34-45, 1975.
25. Thomas ET: Circulatory collapse following succinylcholine: Report of a case. *Anesth Analg 48*:333-337, 1969.
26. Grob D, Namba T, Feldman DS: Alterations in reactivity to acetylcholine in myasthenia gravis and carcinomatous myopathy. *Ann NY Acad Sci 135*:247-275, 1966.
27. Bhala RP: Electromyographic evidence of lower motor neuron involvement in hemiplegia. *Arch Phys Med Rehabil 50*:632-641, 1969.
28. Krueger KC, Waylonis GW: Hemiplegia: Lower motor neuron electromyographic findings. *Arch Phys Med Rehabil 5*: 360-364, 1973.
29. Kakebe K, Narayan MG, Kukulka C, Basmajian JV: Slowing of nerve conduction velocity in hemiplegia: Possible factors. *Arch Phys Med Rehabil 56*:285-289, 1975.

30. Caccia MR, Ubiali E, Schieroni F: Axonal excitability and motor propagation velocity of peripheral nerves in patients with acute vascular lesions of the brain. *J Neurol Neurosurg Psychiatr 39*:900–904, 1976.
31. McComas AJ, Sica REP, Upton ARM, Aquilera N: Functional changes in motoneurones of hemiparetic patients. *J Neurol Neurosurg Psychiatr 36*:183–193, 1973.
32. McComas AJ: *Neuromuscular Function and Disorders.* Butterworth, London, pp. 289–294, 1977.
33. Axelsson J, Thesleff S: A study of supersensitivity in denervated mammalian skeletal muscle. *J Physiol (Lond) 149*: 178–193, 1957.
34. Lambert EH, Mulder DW: Electromyographic studies in amyotrophic lateral sclerosis. *Proc Mayo Clin 32*:441–446, 1957.
35. Mulder DW, Lambert EH, Eaton LM: Myasthenic syndrome in patients with amyotrophic lateral sclerosis. *Neurology 9*: 627–631, 1959.
36. Cooperman LH: Succinylcholine induced hyperkalemia in neuromuscular disease. *JAMA 213*:1867–1871, 1970.
37. Weintraub MI, Megahed MS, Smith BH: Myotonic-like syndrome in multiple sclerosis. *NY State J Med 70*:677–679, 1970.
38. Baskett PJF, Armstrong R: Anesthetic problems in multiple sclerosis. *Anaesthesia 25*:397–401, 1970.
39. Kadis LB: Neurological disorders, in *Anesthesia and Uncommon Diseases* (Katz J, Benumof J, Kadis LB, eds.), Saunders, Philadelphia, pp. 495–496, 1981.
40. Siembowicz E: Multiple sclerosis and surgery. *Anaesthesia 31*:1211–1216, 1976.
41. Frost PM: Anaesthesia and multiple sclerosis. *Anaesthesia 26*:104–105, 1971.
42. Gronert GA, Theye RA: Effect of succinylcholine on skeletal muscles with immbolization atrophy. *Anesthesiology 40*: 268–271, 1974.
43. Kerr JH: Tetanus, in *Cecil Textbook of Medicine* (Beeson PB, McDermott W, Wyngaarden JB, eds.), Saunders, Philadelphia, pp. 436–441, 1979.
44. Roth F, Wuthrich H: The clinical importance of hyperkalaemia following suxamethonium administration. *Br J Anaesth 41*:311–316, 1969.

45. Stone WA, Beach TP, Hamelberg W: Succinylcholine—Danger in the spinal-cord-injured patient. *Anesthesiology 32*:168-169, 1970.
46. Brooke MM, Donovon WH, Stolov WC: Paraplegia: Succinylcholine-induced hyperkalemia and cardiac arrest. *Arch Phys Med Rehabil 59*:306-309, 1978.
47. Tobey RE: Paraplegia, succinylcholine and cardiac arrest. *Anesthesiology 32*:359-364, 1970.
48. Wohlfart G: Collateral regeneration from residual motor nerve fibers in amyotrophic lateral sclerosis. *Neurology 7*: 124-134, 1957.
49. Wise RP: Muscle disorders and the relaxants. *Br J Anaesth 35*:558-564, 1963.
50. MacIntosh FC: Formation, storage, and release of acetylcholine at nerve endings. *Can J Biochem Physiol. 37*:343-356, 1959.
51. Orndahl, G, Sternberg K: Myotonic human musculature: Stimulation with depolarizing agents. Mechanical registration of the succinylcholine, succinylmonocholine, and decamethonium. *Acta Med Scand 172*:389:S3-29, 1962.
52. Hodes R: Electromyographic study of defects of neuromuscular transmission in human poliomyelitis. *Arch Neurol Psychiatr 60*:457-473, 1948.
53. Buchthal R, Honcke P: Electromyographical examination of patients suffering from poliomyelitis ant. ac. up to 6 months after acute stage of the disease. *Acta Med Scand 116*:148-164, 1943.
54. Pinelli P, Buchthal F: Duration amplitude and shape of muscle action potentials in poliomyelitis. *Electroencephalogr Clin Neurophysiol 3*:497-504, 1951.
55. Adams RD, Asbury AK: Diseases of the peripheral nervous system, in *Harrison's Principles of Internal Medicine* (Isselbacher KJ, Adams RD, Braunwald E, Petersdorf RG, Wilson JD, eds.), McGraw-Hill, New York, pp. 2027-2079, 1980.
56. Baginsky RG: A case of peripheral polyneuropathy displaying myasthenic EMG patterns (Abstr). *Electroencephalogr Clin Neurophysiol 25*:397, 1968.
57. Manser J: Abnormal responses in Von Recklinghausen's disease (letter). *Br J Anaesth 42*:183, 1970.

58. Magbagbeola JAO: Abnormal responses to muscle relaxant in a patient with Von Recklinghausen's disease (multiple neurofibromitosis) (letter). *Br J Anaesth 42*:710, 1970.
59. Azar I, Turndorf H: An unusual response to d-tubocurarine in a case of severe peripheral polyneuropathy. *Anesthesiology 46*:371-373, 1977.
60. Fergusson RJ, Wright DJ, Willey RF, Crompton GK, Grant IWB: Suxamethonium is dangerous in polyneuropathy. *Br J Med 282*:298-299, 1981.
61. Solandt, DY, Magladery JW: A comparison of the effect of upper and lower motor neurone lesions on skeletal muscle. *J Neurophysiol 5*:373-380, 1942.
62. Gronert GA, Lambert EH, Theye RA: The response of denervated skeletal muscle to succinylcholine. *Anesthesiology 39*: 13-22, 1973.
63. Marshall M: Action of suxamethonium on ptosis due to third nerve palsy. *Br Med J 2*:1116-1117, 1964.
64. Brim VD: Denervation supersensitivity: The response to depolarizing muscle relaxants. *Br J Anaesth 45*:222-226, 1973.
65. Baraka A: Antagonism of succinylcholine-induced contracture of denervated muscles by d-tubocurarine. *Anesth Analg 60*:605-607, 1981.
66. Lee C, Yang E, Katz RL: Focal contracture following injection of succinylcholine in patients with peripheral nerve injury. *Can Anaesth Soc J 24*:475-478, 1977.
67. Kendig JJ, Bunker, JP, Endow S: Succinylcholine-induced hyperkalemia: Effects of succinylcholine on resting potentials and electrolyte distribution in normal and denervated muscle. *Anesthesiology 36*:132-137, 1972.
68. Tobey RE, Jacobsen PM, Kahle CT, Clubb RJ, Dean MA: The serum potassium response to muscle relaxants in neural injury. *Anesthesiology 37*:332-337, 1972.
69. Stone WA, Beach TP, Hamelberg W: Succinylcholine-induced hyperkalemia in dogs with transected sciatic nerves or spinal cords. *Anesthesiology 32*:515-520, 1970.
70. Gasser HS: Contractures of skeletal muscle. *Physiol Rev 10*: 35-109, 1930.
71. Miller J, Lee C: Muscle diseases, in *Anesthesia and Uncommon Diseases* (Katz J, Benumof J, Kadis LB, eds.) Saunders, Philadelphia, pp. 531-562, 1981.

72. Elmqvist D, Thesleff S: A study of acetylcholine induced contractures in denervated mammalian muscle. *Acta Pharmacol Toxicol 17*:84–93, 1960.
73. Jenkinson DH, Nicholls JG: Contractures and permeability changes produced by acetylcholine in depolarized denervated muscle. *J Physiol (Lond) 159*:111–127, 1961.
74. Gronert GA, Theye RA: Pathophysiology of hyperkalemia induced by succinylcholine. *Anesthesiology 43*:89–99, 1975.
75. Mayer RF: Neuromuscular transmission in single motor units in myasthenia gravis. *Muscle Nerve 5*:S46–S49, 1982.
76. Engel AG, Tsujihata M: The motor end plate in myasthenia gravis and in experimental autoimmune myasthenia gravis. A quantitative ultrastructural study. *Ann of NY Acad Sci 274*: 60–79, 1976.
77. Satyamurti S, Drachman DB, Slone F: Blockade of acetylcholine receptors: A model of myasthenia gravis. *Science 187*:955–957, 1975.
78. Cull-Candy SG, Miledi R, Uchitel OD: Diffusion of acetylcholine in the synaptic cleft of normal and myasthenia gravis human endplates. *Nature 286*:500–502, 1980.
79. Drachman DB: Myasthenia gravis. *N Engl J Med 298*:136–142, 1978.
80. Bergmans J, Fannes-Breselow C, Gribomont B: A reassessment of the neurophysiological evidence for a presynaptic defect in myasthenia gravis. *Electromyogr Clin Neurophysiol 16*:337–349, 1976.
81. Cull-Candy SG, Miledi R, Trautmann A, Uchitel OD: On the release of transmitter at normal, myasthenia gravis, and myasthenic syndrome affected human end-plates. *J Physiol (Lond) 299*:621–638, 1980.
82. Albuqueque EX, Warnick JE, Mayer RF, Eldefrawi AT, Eldefrawi ME: Recent advances in the molecular mechanisms of human and animal models of myasthenia gravis. *Ann NY Acad Sci 377*:496–518, 1981.
83. Brown JC, Charlton JE: A study of sensitivity to curare in myasthenic disorders using a regional technique. *J Neurol Neurosurg Psychiatr 38*:27–33, 1975.
84. Elias SB, Appel SH: Acetylcholine receptor in myasthenia gravis: Increased affinity for alpha bungarotoxin. *Ann Neurol 4*:250–252, 1978.

85. Churchill-Davidson HC: Abnormal response to muscle relaxants. *Proc R Soc Med 48*:621-624, 1955.
86. Stanski DR, Lee RG, MacCannell KL, Karr GW: Atypical cholinesterase in a patient with myasthenia gravis. *Anesthesiology 46*:298-301, 1977.
87. Baraka A, Afifi A, Muallem M, Kachachi T, Frayha F: Neuromuscular effects of halothane, suxamethonium, and tubocurarine in a myasthenic undergoing thymectomy. *Br J Anaesth 43*:91-95, 1971.
88. Foldes FF, McNall PG: Myasthenia gravis: A guide for anesthesiologists. *Anesthesiology 23*:837-872, 1962.
89. Grinar DS, Weinreich AI: Anesthesia for transcervical thymectomy in myasthenia gravis. *Anesth Analg 55*:13-17, 1976.
90. Davies DW, Steward DJ: Myasthenia gravis in children and anaesthetic management for thymectomy. *Can Anaesth Soc J 20*:253-258, 1973.
91. Crawford J: A review of 41 cases of myasthenia gravis subjected to thymectomy. *Anaesthesia 26*:513, 1971.
92. Elder BF, Beal H, DeWald W, Cobb S: Exacerbation of subclinical myasthenia by occupational exposure to an anesthetic. *Anesth Analg 50*:383-387, 1971.
93. Blitt CD, Wright WA, Peat J: Pancuronium and the patient with myasthenia gravis. *Anesthesiology 42*:624-626, 1975.
94. Lake CL: Curare sensitivity in steroid-treated myasthenia gravis: A case report. *Anesth Analg 57*:132-134, 1978.
95. Fogdall RP, Miller RD: Neuromuscular effects of enflurane, alone and combined with d-tubocurarine, pancuronium, and succinylcholine, in man. *Anesthesiology 42*:173-178, 1975.
96. Fillmore RB, Herren AL, Pirlo AF: Curare sensitivity in myasthenia gravis (correspondence). *Anesth Analg 57*:515-516, 1978.
97. Bennett EJ, Schmidt GB, Patel KP, Grundy EM: Muscle relaxants, myasthenia, and mustards? *Anesthesiology 46*:220-221, 1977.
98. Weisman SJ: Masked myasthenia gravis. *JAMA 141*:917-918, 1949.
99. Kornfeld P, Horowitz SH, Genkins G, Papatestas AE: Myasthenia gravis unmasked by antiarrhythmic agents. *Mt Sinai J Med 43*:10-14, 1976.

100. Drachman DA, Skom JH: Procainamide—A hazard in myasthenia gravis. *Arch Neurol 13*:316–320, 1965.
101. Rolbin SH, Levinson G, Shnider SM, Wright RG: Anesthetic consideration for myasthenia gravis and pregnancy. *Anesth Analg 57*:441–447, 1978.
102. Jenkins LC, Chang J, Saxton GD: Myasthenia gravis: Anesthetic and surgical management of the patient undergoing thymectomy. *Can Med Assoc J 93*:198–203, 1965.
103. Eaton LM, Lambert EH: Electromyography and electric stimulation of nerves in diseases of motor unit. *JAMA 13*: 1117–1124, 1957.
104. Rooke ED, Eaton LM, Lambert EH, Hodgson CH: Myasthenia and malignant intrathoracic tumor. *Med Clin N Am 44*:977–988, 1970.
105. Simpson JA: Myasthenia gravis and myasthenic syndrome, in *Disorders of Voluntary Muscle* (Walton JA, ed.), Churchill Livingstone, London, pp. 585–624, 1981.
106. Elmqvist D, Lambert EH: Detailed analysis of neuromuscular transmission in a patient with myasthenic syndrome sometimes associated with bronchogenic carcinoma. *Mayo Clin Proc 43*:689–713, 1968.
107. Denny-Brown D, Nevin S: The phenomenon of myotonia. *Brain 64*:1–18, 1941.
108. Brown GL, Harvey AM: Congenital myotonia in the goat. *Brain 62*:341–363, 1939.
109. Lanari A: The mechanism of myotonic contraction. *Science 104*:221–222, 1946.
110. Landau WM: The essential mechanism in myotonia: An electromyographic study. *Neurology 2*:369–388, 1952.
111. Adie WJ, Greenfield JG: Dystrophia myotonica (myotonia atrophica). *Brain 46*:73–127, 1923.
112. MacDermot V: The histology of the neuromuscular function in dystrophia myotonica. *Brain 84*:75–84, 1961.
113. Feldman SA: *Muscle Relaxants.* Saunders, Philadelphia, pp. 99–108, 1973.
114. Baraka A, Haddad C, Afifi A, Baroody M: Control of succinyldichloline-induced myotonia by d-tubocurarine. *Anesthesiology 33*:669–670, 1970.

115. Hook R, Anderson EF, Noto P: Anesthetic management of a parturient with myotonia atrophica. *Anesthesiology 43*: 689-692, 1975.
116. Ravin M, Newmark Z, Saviello G: Myotonia dystrophica, an anesthetic hazard: Two case reports. *Anesth Analg 54*: 216--218, 1975.
117. Muller J, Suppan P: Case report: Anesthesia in myotonic dystrophy. *Anaesth Intensive Care 5*:70-73, 1977.
118. Mudge BJ, Taylor PB, Vanderspek AFL: Perioperative hazards of myotonic dystrophy. *Anaesthesia 35*:492-495, 1980.
119. Bourke TD, Zuck D: Thiopentone in dystrophia myotonica. *Br J Anaesth 29*:35-38, 1957.
120. Kaufman L: Anesthesia in dystrophia myotonica. *Proc R Soc Med 53*:183-188, 1960.
121. Haley FC: Anesthesia in dystrophia myotonia. *Can Anaesth Soc J 9*:270-275, 1962.
122. Thiel RE: The myotonic response to suxamethonium. *Br J Anaesth 39*:815-820, 1967.
123. Talmage EA, McKechnie FB: Anesthetic management of patient with myotonia dystrophica. *Anesthesiology 20*: 717-719, 1959.
124. Cobham IG, Davis HS: Anesthesia for muscle dystrophy patients. *Anesth Analg 43*:22-29, 1964.
125. Cwizewicz-Adamska J, Wilmowska-Pietrnszymska A: Anaesthesiological problems in myotonic syndromes (description of two cases). *Anaesth Resus Int Ther 2*:93-97, 1974.
126. Mitchell MM, Ali HH, Savarese JJ: Myotonia and neuromuscular blocking agents. *Anesthesiology 49*:44-47, 1978.
127. Pappone PA: Voltage-clamp experiments in normal and denervated mammalian skeletal muscle fibers. *J Physiol (Lond) 306*:377-410, 1980.
128. Peper K, Sterz R: Effects of drugs and antibodies on the post-synaptic membrane of the neuromuscular junction. *Ann NY Acad Sci 377*:519-543, 1981.
129. Morley JB, Lambert TF, Kakulas BA: A case of hyperpyrexia with motonia congenita. *Excerpta Med Int Congr Series 295*:543, 1973.
130. Moulds RFW, Denborough MA: Myopathies and malignant hyperpyrexia (letter). *Br Med J 3*:520, 1974.

131. Furniss P: Malignant hyperpyrexia. *Br Med J 1*:92, 1975.
132. Britt BA, Kalow W: Malignant hyperthermia: A statistical review. *Can Soc Anaesth Soc J 17*:293–315, 1970.
133. Geschwind N, Simpson JA: Procainamide in the treatment of myotonia. *Brain 78*:81–91, 1955.
134. Kennedy F, Wolf A: Experiments with quinine and prostigmine in treatment of myotonia and myasthenia. *Arch Neurol Psychiatr 37*:68–74, 1937.
135. Buchthal, F, Clemmensen S: Electromyographical observations in congenital myotonia. *Acta Psychiatr Neurol 16*: 389–403, 1941.
136. Harvey AM: The actions of quinine on skeletal muscle. *J Physiol (Lond) 95*:45–67, 1939.
137. Leyburn P, Walton JA: The treatment of myotonia: A controlled clinical trial. *Brain 82*:81–91, 1959.
138. Wheeler AS, James FM: Local anesthesia for laparoscopy in a case of myotonia dystrophica (correspondence). *Anesthesiology 50*:169, 1979.
139. Munsat TL: Therapy of myotonia: A double blind evaluation of diphenylhydantoin, procainamide, and placebo. *Neurology 17*:359–367, 1967.
140. Winters JL, McLaughlin LA: Myotonia congenita: A review of four cases. *J Bone Joint Surg 52*:1345–1350, 1970.
141. McComas AJ, Sica REP, Currie S: An electrophysiological study of Duchenne dystrophy. *J Neurol Neurosurg Psychiatr 34*:461–468, 1971.
142. Ragab AHMF: Motor end-plate changes in mouse muscular dystrophy. *Lancet 2*:815–816, 1971.
143. Jerusalem F, Engel AG, Gomez MR: Duchenne dystrophy II. Morphometric study of motor end-plate fine structure. *Brain 97*:123–130, 1974.
144. Dastur DK, Razzak ZA: Possible neurogenic factor in muscular dystrophy: Its similarity to denervation atrophy. *J Neurol Neurosurg Psychiatr 36*:399–410, 1973.
145. Richards WC: Anaesthesia and serum creatine phosphokinase levels in patients with Duchenne's pseudohypertrophic muscular dystrophy. *Anaesth Intensive Care 1*:150–153, 1972.
146. Rowland LP, Eskenazi AN: Myasthenia gravis with features resembling muscular dystrophy. *Neurology 6*:667–671, 1956.

147. Ross RT: Ocular myopathy sensitive to curare. *Brain 86*: 67-74, 1963.
148. Genever EE: Suxamethonium-induced cardiac arrest in unsuspected pseudohypertrophic muscular dystrophy. *Br J Anaesth 43*:984-986, 1971.
149. Isaacs H, Barlow MB: Malignant hyperpyrexia during anaesthesia: Possible association with subclinical myopathy. *Br J Med J 1*:275-277, 1970.
150. Miller ED, Sanders DB, Rawlingson JC, Berry FA Jr, Sussman MD, Epstein RM: Anesthesia-induced rhabdomyolysis in a patient with Duchenne's muscular dystrophy. *Anesthesiology 48*:146-148, 1978.
151. Oka S, Igarashi Y, Takagi A, Nishida M, Sato K, Nakada K, Ikeda K: Malignant hyperpyrexia and Duchenne muscular dystrophy: A case report. *Can Anaesth Soc J 29*:627-629, 1982.
152. Brownell AKW, Paasuke RT, Elash A, Fowlow SB, Seagram CGF, Diewold RJ, Friesen C: Malignant hyperthermia in Duchenne muscular dystrophy. *Anesthesiology 58*:180-182, 1983.
153. Linter SPK, Thomas PR, Withington PS, Hall MG: Suxamethonium associated hypertonicity and cardiac arrest in unsuspected muscular dystrophy. *Br J Anaesth 4*:1131-1332, 1982.
154. Kelper HM, Singer WD, Reynolds RN: Malignant hyperthermia in a child with Duchenne muscular dystrophy. *Pediatrics 71*:118-119, 1983.
155. Fletcher R, Blennow G, Olsson AK, Ranklev E, Torenbrandt K: Malignant hyperthermia in myopathic child. Prolonged postoperative course requiring dantrolene. *Acta Anaesth Scand 26*:435-438, 1982.
156. Rosenberg H, Heiman-Patterson T: Duchenne's muscular dystrophy and malignant hyperthermia: Another warning (letter). *Anesthesiology 59*:362, 1983.
157. Barnes PK: Masseter spasm following intravenous suxamethonium. A case report. *Br J Anaesth 45*:759-760, 1973.
158. Caseby NG: Muscle hypertonus after intravenous suxamethonium: A clinical problem. *Br J Anaesth 47*:1101-1106, 1975.

159. Donlon JV, Newfield P, Sreter F, Ryan JF: Implications of masseter spasm after succinylcholine. *Anesthesiology 49*: 298-301, 1978.
160. Davies DD: Hypertonic syndrome associated with suxamethonium administration (correspondence). *Br J Anaesth 42*:656, 1970.
161. Lessel S, Kawabara T, Feldman RG: Myopathy and succinylcholine sensitivity. *Am J Ophthalmol 68*:789-796, 1969.
162. Peter JB, Stempel K, Armstrong J: Biochemistry and electron microscopy of mitochondria in muscular and neuromuscular diseases, in *Muscle Diseases* (Walton JN, Cana N, Scarlato G, eds.), Excerpta Medica, Amsterdam, p. 228, 1970.
163. Kalow W: Malignant hyperthermia. *Proc R Soc Med 63*: 178-180, 1970.

4
Succinylcholine-Induced Hyperkalemia

DAVID R. GOLDHILL*
Harvard Medical School, and Shriners Burn Institute, Boston, Massachusetts

J. A. JEEVENDRA MARTYN
Shriners Burn Institute, and Massachusetts General Hospital, Boston, Massachusetts

**Present affiliation*: The London Hospital, London, England

I. INTRODUCTION

Succinylcholine was first described in 1906, being used on paralyzed animals. However, its neuromuscular effect was not recognized until 1949. It was introduced into clinical practice in Europe in 1951, and in the United States in 1952 (1), and since then it has been widely used all over the world. Its advantages of rapid onset and recovery were quickly recognized, and at the time of its introduction, succinylcholine was described as the drug most closely fitting the definition of an ideal muscle relaxant. In the year 1982 to 1983, nearly 2000 kg of succinylcholine was sold in the United States alone. It is administered to about 75% of patients having general anesthesia.

Succinylcholine has been found to possess many disadvantages, including some of the most common and most dangerous side effects in anesthesia (Table 1). Overall, succinylcholine administration is followed by an unpredictable response, and is associated with morbidity and mortality. In some patients, it is absolutely contraindicated.

That succinylcholine is dangerous in certain clinical conditions was realized when cases of cardiac arrest following its administration were reported in burn patients. At first, other factors were implicated, such as vagal stimulation during tracheal

Table 1 Disadvantages of Succinylcholine

1. Morbidity
   A. Muscle pain
2. Unpredictability
   A. Atypical pseudocholinesterase
   B. Tachyphylaxis
   C. Phase II block
3. Contraindications
   A. Possible malignant hyperthermia
   B. Myotonia
   C. Possible hyperkalemic response
4. Other side effects
   A. Cardiac dysrhythmias
   B. Increased intraocular pressure
   C. Increased intragastric pressure
5. Interaction with neuromuscular diseases, e.g., myasthenia gravis, muscular dystrophies

intubation, hypovolemia, or abnormal nutritional and metabolic states. Eventually, it was recognized that hyperkalemia triggered by succinylcholine was the cause of the cardiac arrest. This explanation was not universally accepted because not all burn patients experienced cardiac arrest following the use of succinylcholine, and even those who did often had an uneventful response to succinylcholine on other occasions. Later, it became clear that certain injuries predispose patients toward hyperkalemia and possible cardiac arrest following succinylcholine administration, and that there is a latent period after the injury before this response becomes manifest.

II. PATHOPHYSIOLOGY

Normally, neuromuscular transmission depends on the following sequence of events: Nerve action potential arrives at the neuromuscular junction and releases acetylcholine from the presynaptic nerve terminal. The acetylcholine diffuses across the synaptic cleft and interacts with acetylcholine receptors at the postsynaptic motor end-plate. This increases permeability through the receptors' ion channels, causing depolarization of the membrane and generation of muscle action potential and contraction. The effect of acetylcholine at the postsynaptic membrane is then terminated within milliseconds by the local true cholinesterase. This allows immediate repolarization of the postsynaptic membrane and preparation of the neuromuscular junction for the next nerve action potential and muscle contraction.

Succinylcholine consists of two acetylcholine molecules joined back to back. It is therefore not surprising that it has a depolarizing effect similar to that of acetylcholine at the postsynaptic membrane. In normal muscles, the increased ionic permeability caused by depolarizing agents leads to an efflux of potassium from the cell at the end-plate region. Succinylcholine normally causes a rise of up to 0.5 mEq/L in the serum potassium level without cardiovascular consequences. However, in some neuromuscular disorders, the increase in the serum potassium level is much greater, and it may cause cardiac arrest.

Normally, the area sensitive to acetylcholine is limited to the end-plate of the muscle fiber. However, in disorders such as muscular denervation, upper motor neuron lesions, extensive soft tissue injuries, or burns, acetylcholine receptors form outside the end-plate region (2) and the area of chemosensitivity to acetylcholine expands. Eventually, the entire muscle membrane becomes chemosensitive to acetylcholine. The expansion of chemosensitivity begins 3 or 4 days after denervation and is fully developed within 1 to 3 weeks (3). With increased numbers of acetylcholine receptors, a larger surface area is available to release potassium during depolarization, and thus the affected muscles release increased amounts of potassium following the administration of depolarizing agents (4).

Extrajunctional chemosensitivity may also be the cause of resistance to nondepolarizing muscle relaxants in hemiplegia (5) and burn (6) patients. It has been speculated that as long as the resistance to nondepolarizing muscle relaxants is present, extrajunctional chemosensitivity also exists, and there is the possibility of dangerous release of potassium.

Some authors doubt the above explanation for the hyperkalemia and speculate that direct muscle damage and changes in muscle morphology secondary to poor nutrition and atrophy is the cause for the cardiac arrest in these patients. Still others believe that succinylcholine-induced release of catecholamines rather than potassium is the cause of cardiac arrest (7).

III. HYPERKALEMIA IN CLINICAL PRACTICE

Succinylcholine-induced hyperkalemia has been reported in the following clinical conditions (Table 2).

Table 2 Conditions Associated with Succinylcholine-Induced Hyperkalemia

1. Definite
   A. Thermal injuries
   B. Upper motor neuron lesions
      a. Intracranial
      b. Spinal cord
   C. Tetanus
   D. Lower motor neuron lesions
   E. Major trauma
   F. Long-standing septicemia
2. Possible
   A. Peripheral neuropathies
   B. Closed head injury
   C. Ruptured intracerebral aneurysm
   D. Postradiation
   E. Neuromuscular disorders
      a. Parkinson's disease
      b. Muscular dystrophy
      c. Multiple sclerosis
3. Unlikely
   A. Renal failure
   B. Immobilization

A. Thermal Injury

Patients with thermal injuries, in particular those with electrical burns, sustain major nerve and tissue damage and are therefore susceptible to succinylcholine-induced hyperkalemia. There are no reports of succinylcholine-induced hyperkalemia occurring immediately or within a few days after a burn was sustained. There are, however, many reports of a normal response to succinylcholine administration during the early stage after thermal injury and cardiac arrest in the later stage. Hyperkalemia after succinylcholine administration has been recorded as early as 9 days after a thermal injury and peak response was observed at between 20 and 60 days.

The period of vulnerability to succinylcholine in burn patients coincides with the presence of extrajunctional acetylcholine receptors. This further supports the hypothesis that an association exists between the two phenomena. The extrajunctional chemosensitivity may last many months and possibly several years, even when the patient has already recovered and the burns healed (8).

During the period of peak response about one-quarter of burn patients sustain serum potassium levels above 6 mEq/L. Following that period, the risk declines over an additional period of several months. Although usually the increase in serum potassium is related to the dose of succinylcholine, small doses may also be dangerous (9,10) (Fig. 1).

The more extensive the burn, the more likely it is to be associated with hyperkalemia. However, a third-degree burn over as little as 10% of the body surface area has been associated with serum potassium of over 6 mEq/L. Not all burn patients sustain hyperkalemia following succinylcholine administration, and often even in the presence of significant hyperkalemia no cardiovascular changes occur. However, the risk of cardiac arrest in burn patients appears to be about 10 times greater than in normal subjects.

B. Upper Motor Neuron Lesions

Upper motor neuron lesions are lesions of pyramidal neurons in the motor cerebral cortex or of their axons in the spinal cord.

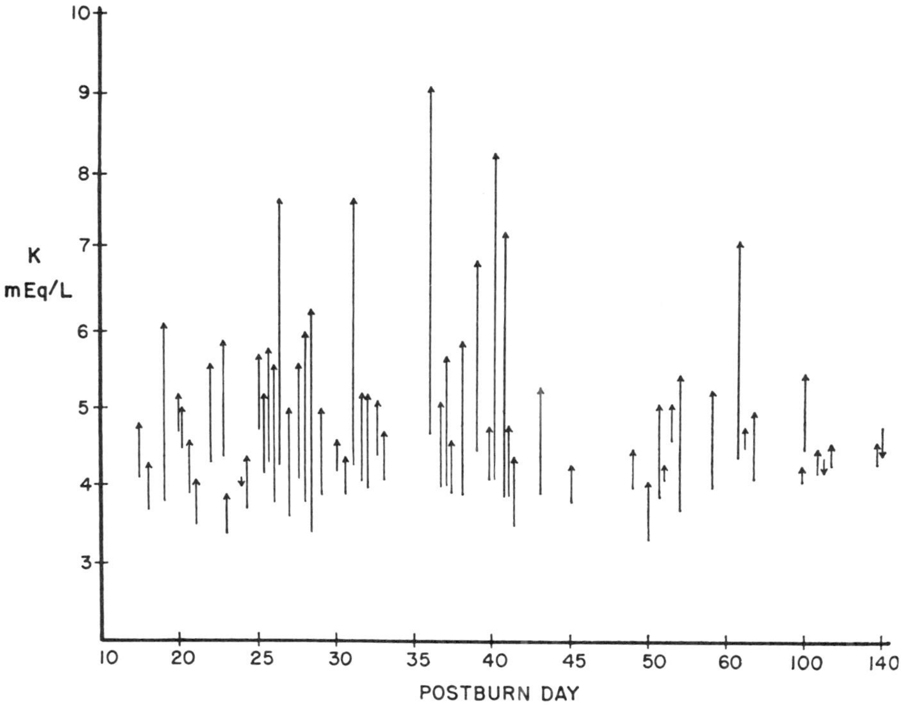

Figure 1 The change in serum potassium level in burned patients after 0.4 mg/kg of succinylcholine. (From Ref. 13, used with permission.)

These lesions have been associated with succinylcholine-induced hyperkalemia (4,11). As with thermal injury, no hyperkalemic response is observed during the immediate postinjury period, although cardiac arrest following succinylcholine administration has been described as early as 7 days following spinal cord injury. Studies in animals demonstrate an increased release of potassium as early as 4 days after the injury and maximum release between 14 and 28 days after the injury. The time to return to normal has not been determined; however, hyperkalemia has been reported to occur as late as 56 days after spinal cord transection (12).

Clinical reports confirm the timing of maximum hyperkalemic response observed in animals. There appears to be a particularly dangerous period at 20-60 days after the injury. However, cardiac arrest following the use of succinylcholine occurred in a paraplegic patient 85 days after the injury, and in a quadriplegic patient 1 year after the injury. In one hemiplegic patient, 18 months after a stroke, the serum potassium level rose 1.5 mEq/L following succinylcholine administration. Since the source of potassium is in the afflicted paralyzed muscles, the greater the bulk of these muscles, the greater the hyperkalemic response.

The hyperkalemia following succinylcholine administration is usually accompanied by characteristic electrocardiographic (EKG) changes. The serum potassium level in blood drawn from the inferior vena cava of paraplegic patients was higher than in blood drawn from the superior vena cava. This suggests that the cause of the hyperkalemia in paraplegic patients is potassium release from the paralyzed muscles below the spinal cord injury (13) (Fig. 2).

C. Tetanus

Tetanus is considered to be an upper motor neuron disorder. Cardiac arrest, probably secondary to succinylcholine-induced hyperkalemia, has been reported in one patient 23 days after the onset of tetanus (14). In another patient, 24 days after the onset of tetanus, the administration of succinylcholine caused a rise in the serum potassium level from 3.8 to 7.4 mEq/L.

D. Encephalitis with Motor Involvement

A patient with a 5-month history of weakness and mental deterioration due to encephalitis had an increase in the serum potassium level from 3.59 to 10.52 mEq/L and hyperkalemic electrocardiographic changes 10 sec after he had received succinylcholine. There were no other cardiovascular changes. The patient, who had been bedridden for a prolonged period of time, had hyperactive tendon reflexes in both arms and in one leg and generalized muscle atrophy (15).

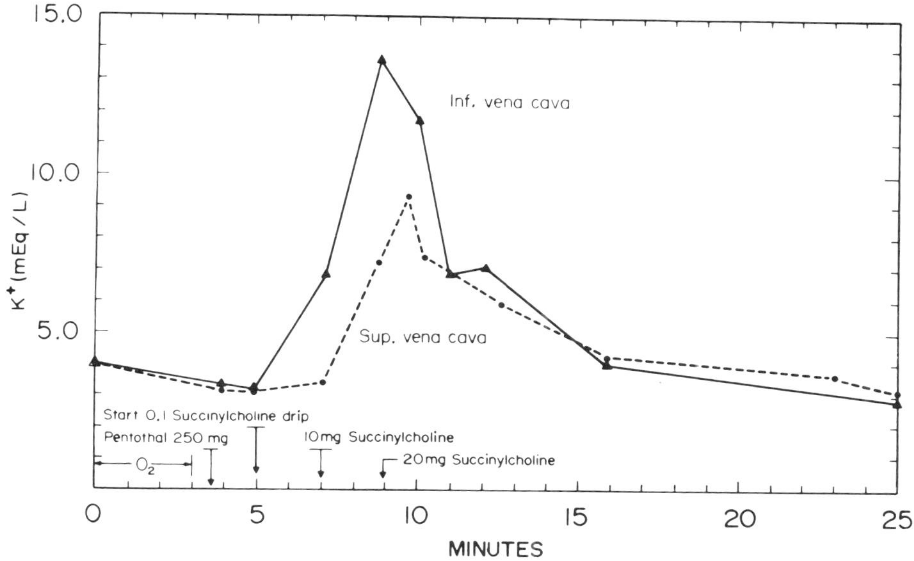

Figure 2 Changes in the serum potassium level in the superior and inferior venae cava in a paraplegic patient during succinylcholine infusion. (From Ref. 13, used with permission.)

E. Lower Motor Neuron Lesions

Lower motor neuron lesions are lesions of neurons at the anterior horn of the spinal cord or of their axons in peripheral nerves. Hyperkalemia following succinylcholine administration has been reported in these patients (4,11). The source of potassium is in paralyzed muscles distal to the neuronal injury. Hyperkalemia has been documented as late as 192 days after a nerve injury.

F. Peripheral Neuropathies

Ventricular fibrillation following succinylcholine administration has been reported in four patients with peripheral neuropathies (16). Although serum potassium levels were not determined, it is likely that hyperkalemia was the cause of the arrhythmias. In one patient with uremic neuropathy, a second dose of succinylcholine caused a significant rise in serum potassium (17).

G. Other Neuromuscular Diseases

1. Parkinson's Disease

There is only one report of electrocardiographic changes and a rise in the serum potassium level following succinylcholine administration in Parkinson's disease. Although physical examination revealed no neurological deficit, the patient had had two previous lumbar laminectomies (18), and this rather than the Parkinsonism could be the possible cause for the hyperkalemia in this patient. In another study, the response of patients with Parkinson's disease was found to be normal (19). The significance of the former report is uncertain.

2. Muscular Dystrophy

Several cases of cardiac arrest following succinylcholine use in patients with muscular dystrophy have been reported, and hyperkalemia was suspected as the cause. In one patient, the hyperkalemia was documented. Myoglobinuria and a rise in creatine phosphokinase (CPK) levels were observed in these patients postoperatively. Since patients with muscular dystrophy are possibly prone to malignant hyperthermia, it seems prudent to avoid the use of succinylcholine in these patients (20).

3. Multiple Sclerosis

There is only one report of hyperkalemia following succinylcholine administration in a patient with multiple sclerosis (20). The degree of rise in the serum potassium level in this case is not clear. There were no cardiovascular changes during the hyperkalemic episode. Other authors have reported normal response to succinylcholine in multiple sclerosis.

H. Major Trauma

Massive trauma has been associated with hyperkalemia and cardiac arrest in patients who received succinylcholine (21). The trauma usually involves extensive soft tissue and bone damage, open wounds, and generalized sepsis. The response to succinylcholine shortly after an injury is normal (22). This is confirmed by the fact that there were no reports of cardiovascular collapse following succinylcholine administration in military hospitals in Viet Nam where soldiers were treated immediately after an injury. On the other hand, there have been several reports of cardiac arrest following the use of succinylcholine in soldiers operated on in military hospitals in the United States 1 to 2 months after the injury had occurred.

The danger of succinylcholine-induced hyperkalemia in trauma patients diminishes gradually as the patients become ambulatory and their wounds heal.

I. Infection

Succinylcholine administration caused a 1.5 mEq/L rise in the serum potassium level of four patients who had had severe postoperative abdominal infection for at least a 2-week duration (23). One of these patients sustained cardiac arrest 3 min after succinylcholine administration, possibly owing to hyperkalemia. Five other patients who had infection for only 9 days or less had a normal response to succinylcholine.

Another study looked at patients with progressive chronic infections such as osteomyelitis or gangrene (24). In these patients, the serum potassium level after succinylcholine administration rose by 0.2–2.3 mEq/L. As in the previous study, the increase in the serum potassium level was directly proportional to the duration of the infection. The degree of hyperkalemia was also related to the severity of the infection and to the duration of bed rest. Bed rest per se has never been associated with succinylcholine-induced hyperkalemia (see Sect. III.J).

J. Immobilization

There are no clinical reports of succinylcholine-induced hyperkalemia secondary to immobilization alone. In dogs with hind limbs immobilized in plaster casts for 29–44 days, muscle atrophy was observed, and following succinylcholine administration there was a slight increase in the serum potassium level. The rise in the serum potassium level was 10 times smaller than the one observed in dogs with chronically denervated muscles (Fig. 3) (25). This refutes the speculation that immobilization per se can cause succinylcholine-induced hyperkalemia (25a).

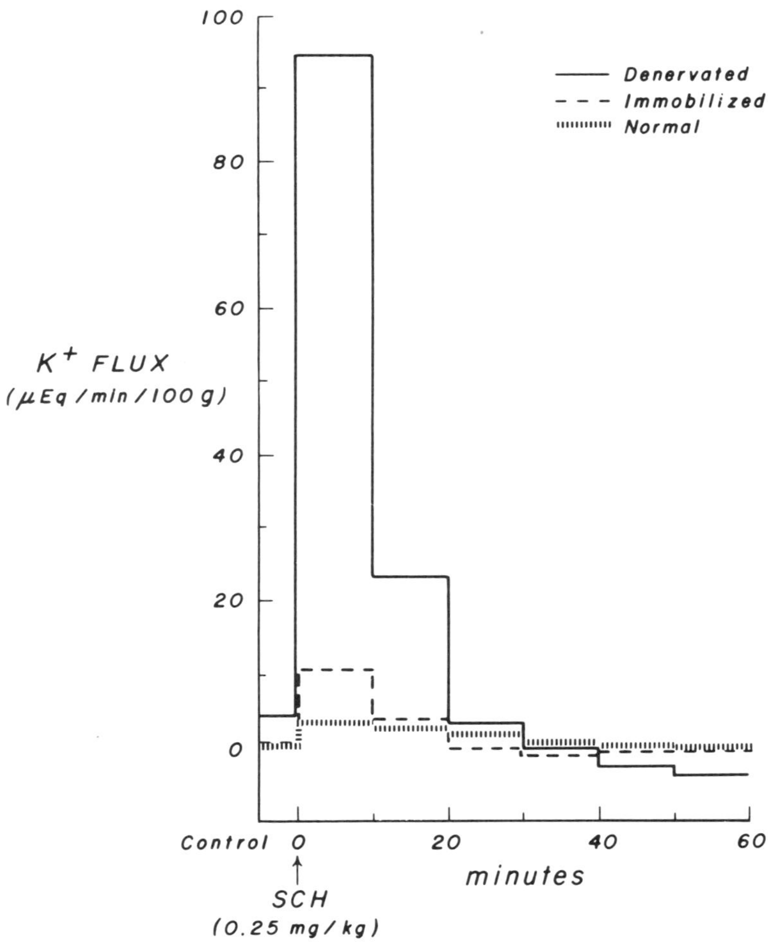

Figure 3 Potassium ions flux from normal, immobilized, and denervated muscles caused by succinylcholine. (From Ref. 25, used with permission.)

K. Closed Head Injury Without Paralysis

Ventricular tachycardia following the use of succinylcholine has been reported in a patient 52 days after he had sustained a closed head injury (26). The patient had no signs of paralysis or muscle denervation. Immediately after tracheal intubation, he developed ventricular tachycardia. Hyperkalemia was suspected, but the serum potassium level was not determined. Eight days later, he was scheduled again for surgery under general anesthesia. This time the serum potassium level was determined before and 4 min after succinylcholine administration, and was found to be 3.8 mEq/L and 6.8 mEq/L, respectively.

L. Ruptured Cerebral Aneurysm

The response to succinylcholine of 22 patients with ruptured (10–15 days old) cerebral aneurysm was studied (27). In four patients, the serum potassium level rose above 6 mEq/L, and the highest value was 10.0 mEq/L. Most patients had no motor deficiencies or muscle paralysis. The authors comment that they have used succinylcholine in about 1000 patients who were scheduled for clipping of cerebral aneurysms and observed no major cardiovascular complications.

M. Muscle Atrophy Secondary to Arterial Insufficiency

Hyperkalemia following succinylcholine administration has been reported in a patient with muscle atrophy secondary to peripheral vascular disease (28). The patient, a 56-year-old man with a 1-year history of an intermittent claudication, was scheduled for revision of an aortic bifurcation graft under general anesthesia. On examination, he had no neurological deficits, but he did have slight atrophy of his right thigh muscles. One minute after receiving succinylcholine, the electrocardiogram showed peaked T waves and ventricular bigeminy. Serum potassium levels, determined in blood samples drawn from the left radial and from the right femoral arteries, were 7.1 and 12.4 mEq/L, respectively. This suggests succinylcholine-induced efflux of potassium from the ischemic muscles of the right leg.

N. Radiation Damage

Radiation therapy may cause hyperkalemia following the use of succinylcholine. A patient with sarcoma who had received radiation therapy sustained cardiac arrest following succinylcholine administration (29). A study of radiation effect on the response of rats to succinylcholine showed no rise in the serum potassium level 1 week after the treatment, but there was a significant rise 3 weeks after the treatment (29).

O. Renal Failure

Several reports have raised the possibility of succinylcholine-induced hyperkalemia in patients with renal failure and uremia. The reports, however, were inconclusive because hyperkalemia was not confirmed by either EKG monitoring or serum potassium determinations. In two patients, abnormally high potassium levels were noted after repeated doses of succinylcholine, but one of the patients had a marked uremic neuropathy, which could possibly be the explanation for the hyperkalemia (17).

Several well-conducted studies found the response to succinylcholine of patients in renal failure to be normal, confirming substantial clinical experience of safe use of succinylcholine in these patients (30,31).

There is still the possibility of a hyperkalemic response in uremic patients due to either repeated doses of succinylcholine or uremic neuropathy. It would seem wise to be circumspect with the use of succinylcholine in renal failure patients, particularly when the serum potassium level is already abnormally high.

IV. COMMON FACTORS IN CLINICAL SITUATIONS

Although the pathophysiology is not always clear, most cases of hyperkalemia following succinylcholine use are associated with a neural or muscular disorder. Evidence, direct and circumstantial, suggests extrajunctional spread of acetylcholine receptors in these disorders, expanding the area from which potassium may be released during depolarization. After a neuromuscular injury, there appears to be a delay from a few days to a week or two before the danger of hyperkalemia develops. In most cases, the danger subsides within 6 months to 1 year after the injury. However, if the disease state is active, the period of risk may be prolonged.

The resistance to nondepolarizing muscle relaxants seen in hemiplegic patients, which apparently is related to extrajunctional acetylcholine receptors, may provide an indicator to identify the patients at risk of hyperkalemic response to succinylcholine: As long as the hemiplegic patient is resistant to nondepolarizing muscle relaxants there exists, presumably, the danger of excessive release of potassium following succinylcholine administration.

The release of potassium following the use of succinylcholine in susceptible patients is abrupt. Serum potassium reaches its peak 2-5 min after succinylcholine administration and it returns to normal within 15-20 min. The degree of rise in the serum potassium level is related to the extent of injury, although dangerous rises in serum potassium have been reported with small burns or minor muscle denervations. The degree of rise in the serum potassium level is probably also related to the total dose of succinylcholine, although cardiac arrest has been reported in an adult patient following only 20 mg of succinylcholine.

V. EKG CHANGES

Characteristic changes that might be seen with an abrupt increase in the serum potassium level are peaking T waves and widening QRS complexes followed by ventricular arrhythmias and fibrillation (Fig. 4). Although peaking of T waves may be seen at a serum potassium level as low as 6 mEq/L, it is not until the level reaches 8 mEq/L or more that the EKG becomes consistently diagnostic of hyperkalemia. Cardiac arrest usually occurs at a serum potassium level of 8 mEq/L or higher, although values of over 11 mEq/L have been recorded without cardiovascular complications. Hyperkalemia per se rarely causes changes in the heart rate or blood pressure, even in the presence of an abnormal EKG, until cardiac arrest occurs. High levels of serum potassium, therefore, may go unnoticed.

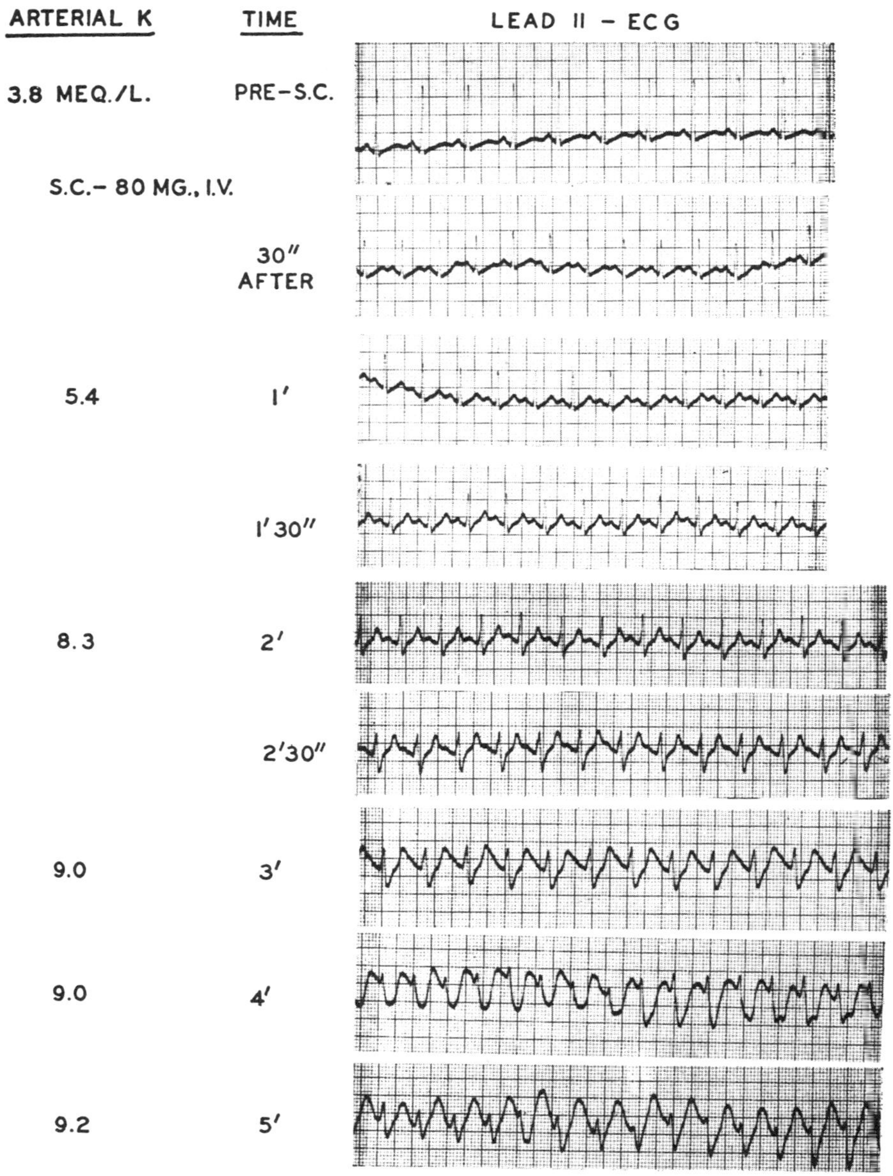

Figure 4 The electrocardiogram and serum potassium levels after succinylcholine (SC) administration in a patient with 1-month-old massive trauma. (From Mazze RI, Dunbar RW: Intralingual

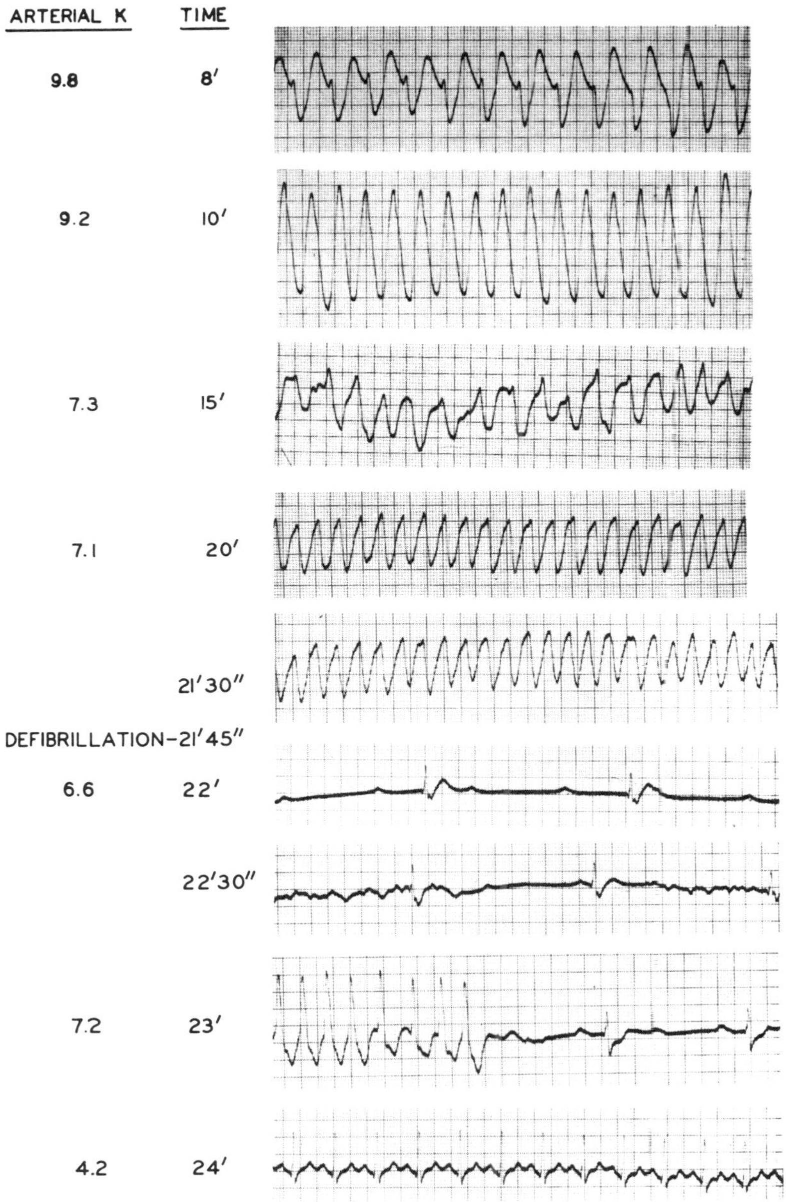

succinylcholine administration in children: An alternative to intravenous and intramuscular routes? *Anesth Analg 47*:605, 1968.)

VI. MODIFYING FACTORS

The danger of hyperkalemia may be enhanced in the presence of verapamil, dantrolene, or hypercarbia. Beta-adrenergic blockers and alpha-adrenergic agonists may potentiate the hyperkalemia by blocking reuptake of potassium by the cells. Also, factors that increase cardiac irritability or alter the level of circulating catecholamines may increase the danger of cardiac arrest in the presence of hyperkalemia.

Various methods have been suggested to reduce the hyperkalemic response to succinylcholine. These include pretreatment with hexafluorenium, diazepam, magnesium sulfate, small doses of succinylcholine (self-taming), or small doses of nondepolarizing muscle relaxants. Although some success has been claimed with these methods, none has been shown to reliably prevent hyperkalemia in patients at risk, and therefore, they are not recommended.

VII. CONCLUSIONS

Although only a few of the patients at risk of hyperkalemia sustain cardiac arrest following succinylcholine administration, the consequences of using succinylcholine in any individual patient are unpredictable. The following clinical disorders are commonly associated with hyperkalemia and cardiac arrest following the use of succinylcholine and this muscle relaxant should not, therefore, be used in these patients:

Burns of any degree or nature
Lower motor neuron lesions
Upper motor neuron lesions
Severe soft tissue and bony injury
Long-standing septicemia

Although the use of succinylcholine in the early stages of these disorders is probably safe, the exact risk period is ill defined. The period of maximum risk is 8 to 10 weeks after the injury, but cardiac arrest has been reported over 6 months after the injury. It is recommended to avoid the use of succinylcholine in these patients. At Shriners Burns Institute in Boston, the practice is to completely avoid the use of succinylcholine until at least 2 years after the injury. This policy could reasonably be extended to other patients at risk.

There are several alternatives to the use of succinylcholine in patients at risk of hyperkalemia. In the patient with a full stomach and at risk of aspiration, tracheal intubation can be achieved without muscle relaxants by awake intubation, facilitated with topical anesthesia. If the risk of aspiration does not exist, tracheal intubation can be achieved by the use of deep inhalation anesthesia or by the administration of one of the nondepolarizing muscle relaxants. Particularly useful for this purpose are the new medium-acting duration muscle relaxants, atracurium and vecuronium. They provide adequate paralysis for intubation with minimal cardiovascular effects, and they are reversible within 30 min after the administration of an intubating dose.

ACKNOWLEDGMENT

Supported in part by grants from the Shriners Burn Institute, Harvard Medical School, Boston, Massachusetts, and the National Institutes of Health, Bethesda, Maryland, GM 21700 and 31569.

REFERENCES

1. Durant NN, Katz RL: Suxamethonium. *Br J Anaesth 54*: 195, 1982.
2. Fambrough DM: Control of acetylcholine receptors in skeletal muscle. *Physiol. Rev 59*:165, 1979.
3. Thesleff S: Effects of motor innervation on the chemical sensitivity of skeletal muscle. *Physiol Rev 40*:734, 1960.
4. Gronert GA, Theye RA: Pathophysiology of hyperkalemia induced by succinylcholine. *Anesthesiology 43*:89, 1975.
5. Moorthy SS, Hilgenberg JC: Resistance to non-depolarizing muscle relaxants in paretic upper extremities of patients with residual hemiplegia. *Anesth Analg 59*:624, 1980.

6. Martyn JAJ, Szyfelbein SK, Ali HH, Matteo RS, Savarese JJ: Increased d-tubocurarine requirements following major thermal injury. *Anesthesiology 52*:352, 1980.
7. Nigrovic V: Succinylcholine, cholinoceptors and catecholamines: Proposed mechanism of early adverse haemodynamic reactions. *Can Anaesth Soc J 31*:382, 1984.
8. Steinbach JH: Neuromuscular junctions and α-bungarotoxin binding sites in denervated and contralateral cat skeletal muscles. *J Physiol 313*:513, 1981.
9. Schaner PJ, Brown RL, Kirskey TD, Gunther RC, Ritchey CR, Gronert GA: Succinylcholine-induced hyperkalemia in burned patients. 1. *Anesth Analg 48*:764, 1969.
10. Gronert GA, Dotin LN, Ritchey CR, Mason AD: Succinylcholine-induced hyperkalemia in burned patients. 2. *Anesth Analg 48*:958, 1969.
11. Smith RB: Hyperkalemia following succinylcholine administration in neurological disorders: A review. *Can Anaesth Soc J 18*:199, 1971.
12. Stone WA, Beach TP, Hamelberg W: Succinylcholine-induced hyperkalemia in dogs with transected sciatic nerves or spinal cords. *Anesthesiology 32*:515, 1970.
13. Tobey RE: Paraplegia, succinylcholine and cardiac arrest. *Anesthesiology 32*:359, 1970.
14. Roth F, Wuthrich H: The clinical importance of hyperkalemia following suxamethonium administration. *Br J Anaesth 41*:311, 1969.
15. Cowgill DH, Mostello LA, Shapiro HM: Encephalitis and a hyperkalemic response to succinylcholine. *Anesthesiology 40*:409, 1974.
16. Fergusson RJ, Wright DJ, Willey RF, Crompton GK, Grant IWB: Suxamethonium is dangerous in polyneuropathy. *Br Med J 1*:298, 1981.
17. Walton JD, Farman JV: Suxamethonium hyperkalemia in uraemic neuropathy. *Anaesthesia 28*:666, 1973.
18. Gravlee GP: Succinylcholine-induced hyperkalemia in a patient with Parkinson's disease. *Anesth Analg 59*:444, 1980.
19. Cooperman LH: Succinylcholine-induced hyperkalemia in neuromuscular disease. *JAMA 213*:1867, 1970.

20. Henderson WAV: Succinylcholine-induced cardiac arrest in unsuspected Duchenne muscular dystrophy. *Can Anaesth Soc J 31*:444, 1984.
21. Birch AA, Mitchell GD, Playford GA, Lang CA: Changes in serum potassium response to succinylcholine following trauma. *JAMA 210*:490, 1969.
22. Kopriva C, Ratliff J, Fletcher JR, Van Tassel P, Stout R: Serum potassium changes after succinylcholine in patients with acute massive muscle trauma. *Anesthesiology 34*:246, 1971.
23. Kohlschutter B, Bauer H, Roth F: Suxamethonium-induced hyperkalemia in patients with severe intra-abdominal infections. *Br J Anaesth 48*:557, 1976.
24. Khan TZ, Khan RM: Changes in serum potassium following succinylcholine in patients with infections. *Anesth Analg 62*: 327, 1983.
25. Gronert GA, Theye RA: Effect of succinylcholine on skeletal muscle with immobilization atrophy. *Anesthesiology 40*: 268, 1974.
25a. Gronert GA, Lambert EH, Theyre RA: The response of denervated skeletal muscle to succinylcholine. *Anesthesiology 39*:13–22, 1973.
26. Stevenson PH, Birch AA: Succinylcholine-induced hyperkalemia in a patient with a closed head injury. *Anesthesiology 51*:89, 1979.
27. Iwatsuki N, Kuroda N, Keisuke A, Iwatsuki K: Succinylcholine-induced hyperkalemia in patients with ruptured cerebral aneurysms. *Anesthesiology 53*:64, 1980.
28. Rao TLK, Shanmugam M: Succinylcholine administration—Another contraindication? *Anesth Analg 58*:61, 1979.
29. Cairoli VJ, Ivankovich AD, Vucicevic D, Patel K: Succinylcholine-induced hyperkalemia in the rat following radiation injury to muscle. *Anesth Analg 61*:83, 1982.
30. Koide M, Waud BE: Serum potassium concentrations after succinylcholine in patients with renal failure. *Anesthesiology 36*:142, 1972.
31. Powell DR, Miller R: The effect of repeated doses of succinylcholine on serum potassium in patients with renal failure. *Anesth Analg 54*:746, 1975.

5

Malignant Hyperthermia

HENRY ROSENBERG and JEFFREY E. FLETCHER
Hahnemann University School of Medicine, Philadelphia, Pennsylvania

I. INTRODUCTION

Malignant hyperthermia (MH) is a muscle disorder associated with extreme elevation in body temperature and often a fatal outcome. Malignant hyperthermia is of great interest to anesthesiologists because of its association with certain anesthetic agents. However, the diagnosis and treatment of this syndrome is also of importance to internists, surgeons, and in particular to intensivists, who occasionally care for MH patients in critical care units. This chapter is an overview of the present state of knowledge of the pathophysiology and clinical, diagnostic, and therapeutic aspects of MH.

II. HISTORY

"Heat stroke" in the operating room was described 70 years ago (1) and was blamed on the lack of temperature control and increased sympathetic stimulation under ether or cyclopropane anesthesia. As we know it today, MH was first recognized and reported by the Australian internist Denborough (2,3). Denborough, who was interested in inherited diseases, suggested that MH is a hereditary disorder, consistent with autosomal dominant inheritance. The awareness of MH was especially raised in the 1950s when potent triggering agents, halothane and succinylcholine, were introduced into the practice of anesthesia, causing a rapid increase in the incidence of MH episodes.

A large gene pool for MH exists in Wisconsin and in Ontario, Canada. Local investigators, therefore [Locher in Wisconsin, and Britt et al. in Ontario (4,5)], have been particularly interested in this syndrome. They traced familial relationships and collected clinical and genetic information, and described the clinical and laboratory variations of MH.

Of special importance to MH research was the discovery of the porcine stress syndrome (PSS). This syndrome resembles MH, and therefore, the PSS-susceptible pig has become the animal model for MH research (6,7).

Kalow et al. (8) were first to describe the increased contracture response to caffeine and/or halothane of muscle biopsy specimens taken from MH patients. Their observations have formed the basis for the most widely used diagnostic test for MH. Using this test on family members of patients with MH has made it possible to prove that MH is a pharmacogenetic disorder of skeletal muscles.

As a result of 25 years of research and clinical experience, a marked decline has occurred in the MH mortality rate, from 70% in the 1960s to about 10% in the 1980s (9,10).

III. EPIDEMIOLOGY AND INCIDENCE

Cases of MH have been reported from most countries where modern anesthesia is practiced (Table 1). The incidence of MH, however, has been difficult to determine for the following reasons:

Table 1 The Incidence of Different Forms of MH in Relation to Type of Anesthesia

	Fulminant	Abortive	Overall
All anesthetics	1:251,063	1:17,435	1:16,303
All general anesthetics	1:211,811	1:15,404	1:14,403
All inhalation anesthetics	1:84,488	1:6,653	1:6,167
with succinylcholine	1:61,961	1:4,506	1:4,201
with succinylcholine	1:174,597	1:20,541	1:18,379
Anesthesia with succinylcholine (no inhalation agent)	1:140,006	1:8,819	1:8,297

Adapted from Ref. 10.

1. There is no central reporting agency for MH.
2. In questionable cases, the clinical diagnosis of MH is often difficult to make, and even harder to confirm.
3. MH-susceptible patients may remain asymptomatic until a second, third, or even fourteenth anesthetic exposure (11). Cain and Ellis (12) report that 50% of MH-susceptible patients have had anesthesia uneventfully prior to the anesthetic exposure that triggered the acute episode. Brief exposure to triggering agents may not necessarily lead to the clinical syndrome.
4. The symptomatology of MH may vary, being mild in some cases, and devastating in others. MH has several clinical forms, possibly owing to more than one underlying abnormality.
5. The diagnostic test for MH is difficult to apply to large populations.
6. The use of triggering agents varies between countries and indeed within locales. Without exposure to triggering agents MH is not manifest.

The original estimates of the incidence of MH are based on Britt's review (4), which reveals an approximate incidence of one in 50,000 anesthetics in adults and one in 15,000 children, with a relatively large proportion of young males. In a later study from Denmark (10), the incidence of fulminant MH was one in 62,000 anesthetics, when inhalation agents and succinylcholine were used

(Table 1). The incidence is likely to be much higher since most patients do not experience fulminant MH. A study from Britain (14) found three cases of MH in a series of 100,000 anesthetics.

Part of the problem of defining the incidence of MH lies in the difficulty in defining MH itself. A common prodrome of MH is masseter muscle rigidity (MMR) following succinylcholine administration. However, MMR is often either resolved uneventfully or accompanied by mild and questionable symptoms of MH. A retrospective review of over 1200 anesthetics at Boston's Children's Hospital revealed that the incidence of MMR following the use of succinylcholine is one in 80 (15). Since susceptibility of MH following an episode of MMR is 50–60% (16), one may expect one "MH alert" case for every 150 pediatric anesthetics where succinylcholine is used. In the study from Denmark, the overall incidence of MMR (including children and adults) was one in 12,000 anesthetics when succinylcholine was used (10). However, that study depended on the reporting of cases, whereas the Boston study was a review of all cases occurring at that hospital. It seems clear that MMR is much more common in children.

The incidence of MH, and the concern regarding this syndrome in a particular locale, is directly related to the prevalence of the MH gene in that locale as well as the type of anesthetics used there, the mean age of the patient population, and the awareness and alertness of the medical staff to MH.

Cases of fulminant MH are only the tip of an iceberg. Many milder cases go unrecognized. Although the fulminant form is rare, the anesthesiologist must be alert to the possibility of MH and detect its signs as early as possible. At least 8 to 10 deaths a year in the United States are due to MH.

IV. INHERITANCE

MH has been known to be heritable from the earliest descriptions of this syndrome. Denborough and Lovell (2), in their original report of MH, observed that several members of their patient's family had died during surgery with symptoms suggestive of MH. Denborough speculated that MH is an inherited syndrome transmitted by an autosomal dominant gene.

The exact mode of inheritance of MH is difficult to determine because of the variability in clinical expression of this syndrome in susceptible patients (Table 2). Most inheritance studies of MH have been based on medical history and serum creatine phosphokinase (CPK) level determinations in family members of susceptible patients; however, both are notoriously poor determinants of MH susceptibility. Relatives of MH-susceptible patients with an elevated CPK level have a 70% chance of being MH susceptible (17). Relatives with a normal CPK level may also be MH susceptible.

Britt's studies (9) showed that MH susceptibility is transmitted through successive generations, and that the syndrome is found in both males and females. She concurred with Denborough that MH is an inherited disorder transmitted by an autosomal dominant gene. Other studies suggest that it can also be transmitted as a multifactorial, autosomal dominant with variable penetrance (4), and multigenetic (18). Our studies, although limited, support the concept of autosomal dominant inheritance by a single gene.

Screening for MH by using in vitro studies of muscle biopsy, although more accurate than clinical evaluation, is complex and expensive and has not been applied to a great extent to studying inheritance of MH in families. Porcine stress syndrome inheritance studies in pigs have not clarified the issue (19). Both autosomal dominant and recessive patterns have been found.

If MH inheritance is analogous to inheritance of other muscle disorders, then it is possible that MH is inherited differently in

Table 2 Inheritance of MH in 93 Families

	%
Clearly autosomal dominant	38
Possibly autosomal dominant	14
Associated with dominant myopathies	3
Isolated	17
? Recessive (isolated)	21
Insufficient Information	7

Source: After Ref. 17, used with permission.

different families. This may include autosomal dominance, sporadic inheritance, and multifactorial inheritance. A simple and accurate test for MH susceptibility would be useful in elucidating the exact mode of MH inheritance.

V. PATHOPHYSIOLOGY AND ETIOLOGY

Three major scientific developments have contributed to the understanding of MH. The first was the recognition that the MH syndrome is transmitted genetically (2,4,9,15). This finding is significant from a mechanistic standpoint, as it suggests that a single inheritable anomaly might explain the abnormal response to anesthetics. A second development was the discovery of greater sensitivity of skeletal muscles of MH-susceptible patients to halothane and/or caffeine (8,13,16,20,21). Specifically, muscle biopsy specimens taken from MH-susceptible patients exhibit contracture (increase in resting tension) thresholds lower than specimens of normal muscles in the presence of halothane and/or caffeine (Fig. 1). This finding made it possible to diagnose and study MH in vitro.

The third development was the discovery of PSS. This syndrome is seen in several inbred strains of pigs and is usually triggered by stress and characterized by muscle rigidity, high temperature, acidosis, and eventually death. The porcine stress syndrome results in unmarketable, pale, soft, and exudative pork (9,13,22–25). It has been recognized that many similarities exist between human MH and PSS. Particularly important is the fact that PSS, just like MH, is triggered by halothane and succinylcholine. Thus, an ideal animal model has become available for studies of MH.

A. Triggering Agents

Agents that trigger MH have been identified by using PSS-susceptible pigs. Of the many potential triggering agents, halothane and succinylcholine are the most important. Because these two agents are structurally unrelated, they probably trigger MH by two different mechanisms. d-Tubocurarine, a

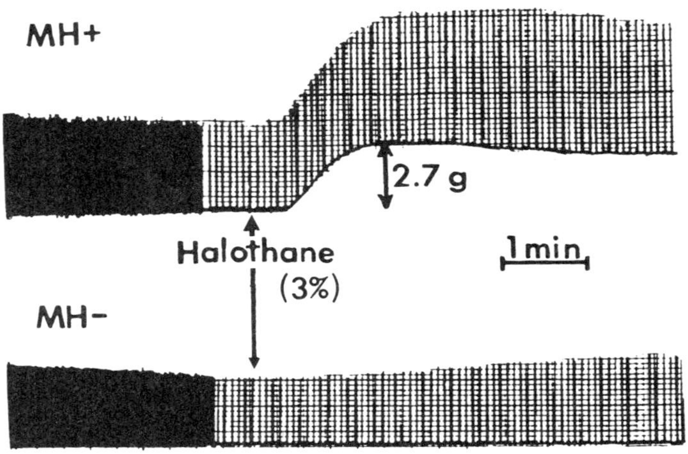

Figure 1 A typical contracture response of a vastus lateralis muscle biopsy specimen taken from an MH-susceptible patient to 3% halothane (upper frame), compared to the response of a similar biopsy specimen taken from a nonsusceptible patient (lower frame). The preparation was stimulated supramaximally at the frequency of 0.2 Hz. Resting muscle tension, 2 g.

nondepolarizing muscle relaxant with an affinity to acetylcholine receptors, antagonizes succinylcholine-induced PSS but not halothane-induced PSS (26,27). It has been speculated, therefore, that acetylcholine receptors play a role in succinylcholine-induced MH. However, a possible common mechanism for triggering agents has become apparent (102).

Although halothane and succinylcholine are the agents most often implicated in MH, most other volatile anesthetic agents may also trigger this syndrome (28). Of the nondepolarizing muscle relaxants, only d-tubocurarine has been implicated in MH (9); however, it does not trigger PSS in pigs (26,27).

B. Phenotypes of MH

Several phenotypes have been reported as a result of outbreeding of PSS pigs. One study has classified three phenotypes by contracture tests and in vivo halothane and succinylcholine challenge (29). Phenotype H is an unequivocal positive based on the in vitro contracture response to halothane 3%. These pigs exhibit PSS when challenged with halothane in vivo. The second phenotype (K) does not exhibit an abnormal contracture response to halothane 3%, but does have a low contracture threshold to caffeine in the presence of halothane and is, therefore, considered an equivocal category. These pigs do not show signs of PSS when challenged in vivo with halothane unless succinylcholine is also administered (29). Even when challenged with halothane and succinylcholine, these pigs do not demonstrate a full-blown PSS episode unless repeatedly challenged or if anesthesia is continued for a prolonged time. The third phenotype (N) is the normal pig. These pigs have no contracture response to halothane 3% in vitro.

The existence of multiple phenotypes in humans is less clear. However, some investigators have reported a spectrum of contracture responses of muscle from MH-susceptible patients, suggesting several phenotypes or different pathophysiologic mechanisms are involved in MH (29,30). Approximately 20% of normal patients would be classified as phenotype K, as determined by the contracture threshold to caffeine with halothane present (31).

C. Role of Catecholamines

Serum catecholamine levels are considerably elevated in both MH and PSS, and it has been proposed that they play an important role in the initiation of these syndromes (33). However, PSS has been shown to occur without an overactive sympathetic nervous system (34). Therefore, it seems unlikely that catecholamines per se can initiate MH. This does not rule out the possibility that catecholamines facilitate the development of acute MH episode from a moderate rise in body temperature to a full-fledged syndrome. Catecholamines stimulate many processes that become active during acute MH. Furthermore, following exercise, serum fatty acids levels in MH patients exceed normal values (35), suggesting increased catecholamine activity.

D. Role of Skeletal Muscles in Thermogenesis

Most investigators believe that the increased thermogenesis in MH is due to a direct effect of halothane or succinylcholine on skeletal muscles, and not on the thermoregulatory center in the brain. In support of this proposal is the increased response in vitro to halothane of muscle biopsy specimens taken from MH patients (8,16,20,21). The increase in whole body oxygen consumption that occurs during an MH episode appears to be entirely due to an increase in muscle oxygen consumption (36).

The heat production in skeletal muscles during an MH episode is believed to be derived from processes stimulated directly or indirectly by an overload of calcium ions. These processes would include aerobic and anaerobic metabolism, hydrolysis of adenosine triphosphate (ATP), and neutralization of hydrogen ion production (5,18).

E. Interaction Between Halothane and Succinylcholine

Halothane and succinylcholine are most often implicated in triggering MH. Clinically, synergism has been observed between the two agents in relation to the incidence of MMR (15), increase in serum CPK activity (37,38), elevation of core temperature (32), and incidence of myoglobinemia (39). A similar in vitro synergism has been observed in relation to muscle contracture (40). The mechanism of this synergism may be linked to phospholipase A_2 activity (102).

F. Role of Calcium

The enhanced metabolism in MH is generally believed to be a result of an abnormally high concentration of myoplasmic calcium ions (41). Studies of total calcium ion content in muscles of MH-susceptible patients have shown either a normal (42) or lower than normal (43) level. However, total cell calcium determination does not reveal the level of free myoplasmic calcium. Using electron microscopy and microprobe analysis, Stadhouders et al. (44) observed a large accumulation of calcium ions in the mitochondria of muscle biopsy specimens taken from pigs during a PSS episode. Recently, the elevated myoplasmic calcium levels have been directly confirmed in humans (104) and pigs using a calcium-selective microelectrode. Also the elevated calcium levels are lowered by dantrolene (61).

The calcium ions in the myoplasm most likely originate in the sarcoplasmic reticulum, and to a lesser degree in the mitochondria. Some may also diffuse in from outside the cell across the sarcolemma. It is likely that the myoplasmic calcium concentration in MH is high because cellular mechanisms, which are responsible for its removal, are either inhibited and/or their capacity to remove calcium from the cell is exceeded.

VI. DIAGNOSIS OF MH

A. Clinical Diagnosis

The perioperative diagnosis of MH may be simple, but on occasion it is frustratingly difficult. Malignant hyperthermia may occur at any time during anesthesia and surgery; however, the syndrome is most likely to occur on induction of anesthesia (especially when succinylcholine is used) or during emergence from anesthesia as muscle tone begins to return.

Malignant hyperthermia may manifest as either a fast rise in metabolism and body temperature or as a slowly progressing process, "picking up steam" with time before it becomes "explosive." The intensity of an MH episode depends on the specific triggering agent, on whether the patient had been exercising prior to the exposure to the triggering agent (45), and on the inherent heterogenicity of MH. In general, when the syndrome is triggered by succinylcholine, the clinical picture tends to be explosive. However, MH has occurred in patients who had had a previous uneventful response to succinylcholine and/or halothane.

A common manifestation of MH, and yet not a specific sign, is MMR or total body rigidity following succinylcholine administration. Britt has estimated that muscle rigidity occurs in about 80% of MH patients under general anesthesia (9). The rigidity lasts a few minutes and is not relieved by additional doses of succinylcholine. Not infrequently, only arrhythmias and slight temperature elevation accompany MMR. If an episode of MMR is not followed by signs of acute MH, dantrolene may be withheld, but these patients should be observed for at least 24 hr because often myoglobinuria, muscle aches, and muscle weakness occur (46).

Because MMR is often transient and uneventful, it is tempting to continue with the anesthesia and surgery. However, the complete syndrome of MH may follow MMR, especially if triggering anesthetic agents are in use (47). Most studies show that 50% or more of patients who develop MMR are confirmed MH-susceptible patients (15,16,29). If anesthesia is discontinued, the patient usually recovers and experiences only myoglobinuria and a rise in the CPK level 6–24 hr later.

The earliest symptoms of MH are tachycardia and tachypnea caused by hypermetabolism and hypercarbia. Since most patients undergoing general anesthesia are paralyzed, tachypnea is usually not seen. Tachycardia is also an unreliable sign because it may be caused by a variety of other factors besides MH, such as light anesthesia, hypovolemia, drug effect, and thyroid crisis (48).

A rise in temperature is the most striking sign of MH; however, it is likely to occur late in the developing syndrome because it depends on an increase in the metabolic rate. Once the temperature starts rising, it is likely to rise in an accelerated fashion of the increase in the metabolic rate. The rise in body temperature may go undetected if the patient had been hypothermic prior to the onset of MH. Attention should be paid to both the absolute and relative changes in body temperature.

B. In Vitro Diagnosis

The most commonly used and accepted diagnostic procedure for MH is the in vitro contracture test of muscle biopsy specimens (49). There are several versions to this test, but the halothane contracture test is regarded as the most sensitive and specific (16,50). The caffeine contracture test is less sensitive, but it is very specific (16,50). The halothane-caffeine contracture test is the most sensitive, but it is least specific (31). The latter detects the phenotype K (29,30), which is a questionable form of MH.

Three other in vitro diagnostic tests for MH have been reported, but they are not generally accepted as reliable. These are the calcium uptake test, the skinned fiber test, and the platelet nucleotide depletion test. A report claiming that muscles from MH patients contain abnormal proteins, as determined by gel electrophoresis (51), has been refuted (52,53). No obvious differences in muscle protein profiles have been found between MH-susceptible patients and normal subjects (54–56). Another noninvasive test entailing study of succinylcholine effect on the patient's electromyogram (EMG) has been reported (57); however, this report is preliminary and can not yet be evaluated. A complete review of MH laboratory tests is available (18).

VII. MANAGEMENT OF ACUTE MH

Malignant hyperthermia therapy consists of symptomatic support and administration of dantrolene, a specific therapeutic agent. In order to be effective, the treatment of acute MH must be planned ahead and implemented promptly and continuously. The earlier the diagnosis is made and the lower the body temperature on initiation of therapy, the better the prognosis (9). Dantrolene as well as a written plan for MH management should be readily available in all anesthetizing locations.

A. Supportive Measures

Once the diagnosis of MH has been made, all potential triggering agents should be discontinued; e.g., inhalation agents (including nitrous oxide) and succinylcholine. The patient should be hyperventilated with oxygen, 100%, at high flow rates in order to satisfy the increased metabolic needs of oxygen uptake and carbon dioxide elimination. If possible, the breathing hoses and the CO_2 absorbent should be replaced with new ones.

In fulminant cases, 2-4 mEq/kg of bicarbonate should be administered to combat metabolic acidosis. In milder cases (arterial $PCO_2 < 60$ mmHg and pH > 7.25), hyperventilation alone is usually sufficient to correct the acidosis. A capnograph should be used in order to monitor continuously the end-tidal CO_2.

Correction of the hyperthermia should be accomplished as quickly as possible by using ice packs for external cooling, and gastric and wound lavage with cold saline for internal cooling. Some recommend peritoneal dialysis, and if necessary, even cardiopulmonary bypass to facilitate cooling of the patient. In order to avoid excessive cooling and hypothermia, the cooling efforts should cease when the patient's body temperature is reduced to 38°C.

Fluid and electrolyte imbalance often occurs during acute MH, and it should be corrected and followed even after the symptoms of MH have subsided. In severe cases, rhabdomyolysis may also occur and myoglobin may be released from injured muscles. This should be treated vigorously with diuretics, since myoglobin may precipitate in renal tubuli and cause renal failure.

Hyperkalemia should be managed with dextrose and insulin. However, this may result in hypokalemia. If possible, potassium replacement should be avoided, since it may possibly trigger another MH episode (105).

Hypocalcemia often occurs during treatment of MH, but there is usually no need to correct it.

As soon as treatment of MH has begun, the patient's coagulation profile should be determined in order to detect disseminated intravascular coagulation (DIC). If there are already signs of DIC, the usual management of this syndrome should be implemented.

B. Dantrolene Therapy

Dantrolene was first introduced into medicine as an oral preparation to treat muscle spasticity. In 1979, it was introduced for intravenous use as a specific therapeutic agent for MH. It is highly effective in the treatment as well as the prophylaxis of MH (13,18,58), and it has a high therapeutic index (59).

Dantrolene operates inside the muscle cell by reducing calcium release (58,60) and increasing calcium ion reuptake by the sarcoplasmic reticulum. This reduces the intracellular calcium content (61) and in turn the excitation-contraction coupling at the transverse tubular system of the cell and thereby muscle activation. In vitro, dantrolene prevents halothane-induced contracture of muscle biopsy specimens taken from MH patients (62).

The initial dose of dantrolene for the treatment of an acute episode of MH is 2.5 mg/kg intravenously. This produces a therapeutic level of 2.5 μg/ml in the blood for 2–4 hr (63), with approximately a 12-hr half-life (64). If indicated, this dose may be repeated several times. Although it has been recommended that the total dose of dantrolene should not exceed 10 mg/kg, more may be given if the clinical situation calls for it. Dantrolene is poorly dissolved in saline and is therefore kept lyophilized and mixed with mannitol (each ampule contains 25 mg of dantrolene and 3 g of mannitol). When needed, dantrolene and mannitol are mixed with sterile distilled water.

The best guide and indicator of effective dantrolene therapy is the patient's heart rate. Usually, the heart rate responds promptly to the therapy. If the patient sustains an arrhythmia, it is usually resolved after the acidosis and hyperkalemia are corrected. If necessary, procaine or procainamide, 2–7 mg/kg, may be added to control the arrhythmia.

Acute administration of dantrolene has several side effects, but none are serious. The most common side effect is muscle weakness, which may last for 24 hr after the treatment. Dantrolene has little effect on myocardial contractility, since the heart depends on extracellular calcium. Also, dantrolene has an insignificant effect at the neuromuscular junction, and the response to nondepolarizing muscle relaxants in the presence of this drug is normal. Although dantrolene-induced hepatitis has been reported, it occurs only following long-term therapy (58).

Calcium-channel blockers have been recommended in the management of MH (65–67); however, because of interaction with dantrolene, they may cause significant cardiac depression (65,67, 68) and life-threatening hyperkalemia. Furthermore, some report failure of calcium blockers in preventing and treating MH (65) or PSS (69,70).

C. Laboratory Follow-Up

The initial laboratory findings during an episode of MH are increased oxygen consumption and carbon dioxide production (71). If ventilation is maintained at a constant level, the end-tidal CO_2 would rise abruptly by two- to three-fold. Similar changes would occur in arterial PCO_2 and pH. Gronert believes that if in the presence of constant ventilation, the arterial PCO_2 rises above 60 mmHg and the base excess is negative and $>$ 6 mEq, then the patient is probably developing acute MH. If the patient had been hyperventilated prior to the onset of acute MH, then the arterial PCO_2 may not reflect the hypermetabolic state of the patient. That is why venous as well as arterial PCO_2 determinations are recommended during an acute MH episode.

A rise in the serum CPK level is a characteristic of MH, the determination of which may be helpful confirming a questionable case of MH. We have recently reported that a rise in the CPK level to over 20,000 IU following an episode of MMR indicates MH susceptibility (103) (Table 3). Although normally the CPK level rises 10 to 15-fold after most surgical procedures (38), a typical rise in the CPK level following acute MH is 40 to 100-fold. Creatine phosphokinase levels of over 100,000 IU have been observed in some MH patients following an acute episode. However, it may take 6-24 hr after an hyperthermic episode before serum CPK starts to rise. This test, therefore, is not useful during the acute stage of MH.

Table 3 Changes in CPK Level Following Succinylcholine Administration in MH and non-MH Patients with a History of MMR

		MH patients	Non-MH patients
Age (yr)		11.9 + 1.5	10.3 + 1.2
Sex	M	19	15
	F	20	23
CPK changes	M (17)	8094 + 3287	5917 + 1346
	F (13)	15,190 + 4835	4412 + 1040

Adapted from Ref. 103.

Myoglobinuria usually occurs when the CPK level exceeds 15,000 IU. Urine and blood may be analyzed for myoglobin using immunological tests. A rapid screening test can be achieved if a hemastix is positive in the absence of microscopic red cells.

Other enzymes such as lactic acid dehydrogenase, transaminases, and aldolase may also be elevated in fulminating MH (72). Hyperkalemia occurs owing to potassium release from the liver (73). The release of enzymes and potassium from the liver is probably due to hepatocellular damage caused by the high temperature and the acidosis that accompany acute MH.

Disseminated intravascular coagulation may occur during the acute stage of MH, probably as a result of thromboplastins released by the high temperature, shock, and free membranes released by destroyed cells. If bleeding diathesis develops, the platelet count, prothrombin time, partial thromboplastin time, and fibrinogen level should be determined.

We have recently reviewed the clinical manifestations in about 250 patients who had previously had muscle biopsy specimens studied for MH (H. Rosenberg and J. Fletcher; unpublished data). About 50% of the patients were referred for muscle biopsy because they had had an episode of MMR during induction of anesthesia. Of the 250 patients in the study, 101 were proven to be MH susceptible. Of those patients who had a concurrent rise in temperature, muscle rigidity, and an elevated CPK level, 67% had positive contracture studies for MH. Of those patients who had clinical symptoms suggestive of MH, two-thirds had had a history of muscle cramps.

D. Management of Recrudescence

Recrudescence of MH, although uncommon, may occur up to 36 hr following a fulminant episode of MH. This may occur despite adequate initial dantrolene therapy (13). Arterial and venous blood gases should be determined periodically after an episode of acute MH, and the bladder should be catheterized for urinary output monitoring. The serum CPK and potassium levels and the acid-base status as well as vital signs should be assessed periodically.

There are no good guidelines for dantrolene therapy after the resolution of an acute episode of MH. In severe cases, it seems prudent to continue dantrolene therapy with 1–2 mg/kg every 4–6 hr for at least 24 hr. Some recommend switching to oral dantrolene, 4 mg/kg a day for 4–5 days. Muscle weakness due to damage caused by the hyperthermia and a direct depressing effect of dantrolene may occur after an MH episode and may require supportive measures (46).

VIII. MANAGEMENT OF SUSCEPTIBLE PATIENTS

Malignant hyperthermia-susceptible patients and their relatives require special anesthetic care. Although some controversy surrounds this issue, there is a consensus on the basic principles of management.

A. The Preoperative Interview

A complete history of previous episodes of MH in the patient and, if pertinent, in relatives of the patient should be taken. The presence of a myopathy and other muscle disorders such as strabismus, muscle cramps, scoliosis, and hernias should be evaluated and documented. In general, patients have become more aware of the anesthetic risk of this syndrome and frequently present the anesthesiologist with many questions regarding the risk of anesthesia. The patient should be reassured that the danger of MH is significantly reduced when the physician anesthesiologist is aware of the patient's susceptibility.

Since anxiety may possibly play a role in triggering MH, it is recommended that verbal reassurance and anxiolytic drugs be used to alleviate preoperative anxiety in these patients.

B. Premedication

Narcotics, benzodiazepines, ataractics, barbiturates, and antihistamines are believed to be safe for MH-susceptible patients. Phenothiazines should be avoided for a reason given in Section VIII.G of this chapter. Although anticholinergic agents have been implicated in MH (9), the evidence is largely anecdotal. We have given atropine to MH-susceptible patients in combination with an anticholinesterase for reversal of nondepolarizing muscle relaxants without incident (74).

C. Preoperative Administration of Dantrolene

Except when scheduled for diagnostic muscle biopsy, MH-susceptible patients should be treated with intravenous dantrolene preoperatively (75). By studying the response of PSS-susceptible pigs, the prophylactic dose of dantrolene for MH patients was determined to be 2.5 mg/kg. It should be given over a 15–30-min period shortly before surgery. Prophylactic oral dantrolene is not recommended.

D. The Anesthesia Machine

There is no clear evidence that traces of halothane may trigger MH. It seems prudent, however, to use an anesthesia machine that has never been exposed to volatile anesthetic agents for MH-susceptible patients. If such a machine is not available, the following guidelines are recommended for machine preparation:

1. Use a new disposable anesthesia breathing circuit.
2. Drain and disconnect the vaporizers.
3. Change the carbon dioxide absorbent.
4. Turn the oxygen flowmeter on at the rate of 3–5 L/min for 12–24 hr.

E. Monitoring

Since the earliest metabolic change during MH reaction is an increase in carbon dioxide production, continuous end-tidal CO_2 monitoring by capnography is recommended during general anesthesia in these patients. If a capnograph is not available, blood gases should be analyzed periodically for arterial and venous PCO_2.

Body temperature should be monitored at the nasopharynx, rectum, or esophagus. The reliability of skin or urinary temperature monitoring in MH patients has not been established (76).

F. Anesthetic Management

Whenever anesthesia, general or regional, is contemplated in an MH-susceptible patient, 36 ampules of dantrolene should be available in the operating room and access to additional dantrolene should be assured. Given the shelf life of dantrolene (3 years) and the cost of 36 ampules (under $2000), stocking this drug is not an unreasonable precaution. An ice-making machine and a refrigerator containing several liters of cold intravenous solutions should also be in close proximity.

Because of their well-established safety, the preferred anesthetic techniques for MH-susceptible patients are regional and local nerve blocks. We feel that ester- as well as amide-type local anesthetics are safe in MH susceptibles (77,78).

If general anesthesia cannot be avoided, induction with sodium pentothal followed by nitrous oxide–oxygen, pancuronium, and a narcotic is recommended. Other induction agents that are considered safe are midazolam (78), diazepam, droperidol, and althesin (13). For additional information on the safety of anesthesic adjuvants in MH, see Section VIII.G in this chapter.

Controversy surrounds the use of nitrous oxide in MH-susceptible patients. There are two reports of MH associated with nitrous oxide, one in a dental patient (18), and the other in a patient who developed acute MH during nitrous oxide–narcotic anesthesia despite pretreatment with intravenous dantrolene (79). Since there are no other reports of MH associated with this commonly used anesthetic gas, at worst, nitrous oxide has a weak MH-triggering effect (80).

G. Safety of Anesthetic Adjuvants

We believe that MH can be triggered only by pharmacological agents. While there is consensus on the safe use of many anesthetic agents and adjuvants in MH, there is still controversy about many others (Table 4). The following is the present state of knowledge regarding the safety of commonly used anesthetic adjuvants.

Table 4 Selection of Anesthetic Agents and Adjuvants for MH Patients

Safe	Avoid
Barbiturates, pancuronium	Volatile anesthetic agents
Ester-type local anesthetics	Potassium chloride
Narcotics (except meperidine)	Succinylcholine
Atracurium	
	Unsettled
Use with care	Catecholamines
d-Tubocurarine	Anticholinergics
Nitrous oxide	Anticholinesterases, digitalis
Phenothiazines	

1. Nondepolarizing Muscle Relaxants

Nondepolarizing muscle relaxants such as d-tubocurarine and pancuronium attenuate the onset and severity of PSS (81). In man, clinical experience indicates that pancuronium is safe (13,18), although several questionable reports implicate this muscle relaxant as a triggering agent. The clinical experience with other nondepolarizing muscle relaxants is limited. Atracurium is safe in PSS and MH (82). A recent study on the use of vecuronium in PSS was inconclusive (83): One out of six susceptible pigs developed PSS. It is possible that stress rather than vecuronium triggered PSS in that one pig.

2. Anticholinesterases

It has been speculated that anticholinesterases could possibly trigger MH by depolarizing the neuromuscular junction. However, our experience suggests that reversal of nondepolarizing muscle relaxants with an anticholinesterase in combination with an anticholinergic agent is safe (74).

3. Phenothiazines

Phenothiazines trigger neuroleptic malignant syndrome (NMS), a syndrome that has been associated with MH (84,85). In vitro, phenothiazines cause contracture of muscle biopsy taken from MH patients, and increase intracellular calcium concentration (86). Phenothiazines, therefore, are contraindicated in MH-susceptible patients.

4. Local Anesthetics

Procaine, an ester-type local anesthetic, has been reported to antagonize PSS (26) and MH (87); however, these observations are controversial (88). In vitro, procaine blocks halothane-induced (89) and caffeine-induced (63) contractures and is probably safe to use in susceptible patients. Procainamide antagonizes caffeine-induced contracture; however, excessive doses are required, which may cause side effects. Ester-type local anesthetic agents, therefore, are safe but have no apparent use in preventing or treating MH.

Lidocaine, an amide-type local anesthetic, increases halothane-induced (89) and caffeine-induced (90) contractures in vitro. However, in vivo, it triggers neither PSS (91,92) nor MH (77).

5. Ketamine

There are on one hand reports that ketamine triggers MH, and on the other that it is safe in PSS (13). Ketamine should probably be avoided in MH-susceptible patients because it normally causes a slight rise in body temperature, and this may complicate the diagnosis of acute MH in susceptible patients.

6. Catecholamines

The relation of catecholamines and sympathetic system activity to MH is not clear. Hall et al. (93) reported that PSS is triggered in susceptible pigs by sympathetic agonists, particularly alpha-adrenergic agents, and that adrenalectomy protects against PSS. In contrast, Gronert (34) could not trigger MH in susceptible swine with either alpha or beta agonists.

Although a rise in the catecholamines level during an acute MH episode has been reported, this is apparently a result rather than the cause of MH. Sympathetic denervation by spinal anesthesia did not delay the onset of halothane-induced MH, although the blood catecholamine level did not rise during the acute episode. We believe that when necessary, vasopressors can be used in MH-susceptible patients.

H. The Postoperative Period

If an MH-susceptible patient shows no signs of MH during general anesthesia, postoperative dantrolene therapy is not necessary. However, the patients should be observed closely for at least 4–6 hr postoperatively. We know of no postoperative incidents of acute MH in patients who were treated prophylactically with dantrolene before surgery, provided appropriately safe anesthetic agents and adjuvants were used.

I. The Obstetrical Patient

Contrary to statements in the literature, we are not convinced that the stress of labor may precipitate acute MH in susceptible patients. However, since regional anesthesia has been shown to be safe in these patients, an epidural block is recommended for labor and delivery.

Prophylactic dantrolene administration in the MH-susceptible obstetrical patient is of special concern because of possible effects of this drug on the fetus. The fetal to maternal dantrolene blood level ratio is probably 0.4 (94). Prophylactic administration of dantrolene to obstetrical patients is therefore not recommended. However, body temperature and other vital signs should be monitored closely during labor and delivery.

IX. PREVENTION

In view of the devastating nature of MH, preparations should be made not only to treat the acute syndrome as early as possible but also to prevent its occurrence.

Prevention begins with a thorough preoperative interview of all surgical patients. In addition to a personal history of anesthetic exposure, a family history should also be obtained. Fortunately, patients usually volunteer readily information on anesthesia complications in their family. The history should include that of younger members of the family, particularly if any of them required prolonged hospitalization and ventilation following a minor surgical procedure.

Information should also be obtained on neuromuscular disorders in the patient and the family. A variety of nonspecific muscle abnormalities may be more prevalent in MH susceptibles, such as subluxating joints, ptosis, strabismus, scoliosis, and muscle cramps. However, these problems are common in the general population and rarely lead to acute MH. In our experience, nonexertional muscle cramps or significant scoliosis are reasonably good markers of MH susceptibility in a patient with an immediate relative who is a confirmed MH susceptible.

The decision whether to proceed with anesthesia and surgery in a patient who has had an unconfirmed episode of MH, or in a patient with a distant relative who is a confirmed MH susceptible, is difficult. In such cases, it is recommended that the anesthesia team treat these patients as if they were MH susceptible, and that the same precautions be taken (see Sect. VIII in this chapter). Whether muscle biopsy for MH diagnosis should be performed first depends on the nature and urgency of the proposed surgical procedure.

The single best monitor to detect an acute episode of MH at its inception is a capnograph for continuous end-tidal CO_2 determination (95).

X. DISORDERS ASSOCIATED WITH MH

Although MH is clearly a muscle disorder and has been associated with several different myopathies, a cause and effect relationship has not been established. The following muscle disorders have been associated with MH: NMS, central core disease, muscular dystrophy, myotonia, the King-Denborough syndrome, and the Schwartz-Jampal syndrome. Other medical disorders have also been associated with MH: Scoliosis, congenital subluxation of joints, osteogenesis imperfecta, arthrogryposis, neurofibromatosis, Burkitt's lymphoma, sudden infant death syndrome (SIDS), pheochromocytoma, and heat stroke (Table 5).

A. Muscular Dystrophy

Our laboratory has analyzed muscle biopsy specimens from five patients with muscular dystrophy. In three cases, the halothane contracture was similar to that of MH patients (96). Several clinical cases of MH have also been reported in Duchenne muscular dystrophy patients. Some treat muscular dystrophy patients prophylactically with dantrolene; however, this may cause severe muscle weakness. It is recommended that succinylcholine be avoided in these patients and that their body temperature and other vital signs be closely monitored during the perioperative period. It is not known whether other dystrophies are associated with MH.

B. Myotonia

It is well established that succinylcholine causes muscle contracture in myotonic patients (97). However, only a few cases of myotonia associated with MH have been reported (18). We have confirmed MH susceptibility in one myotonia congenita patient by using in vitro contracture tests.

C. Neuroleptic Malignant Syndrome

Several researchers have pointed out the similarities between NMS and MH. Dantrolene has been used to treat NMS (98–100);

Table 5 Disorders Associated with MH

Central core myopathies	Osteogenesis imperfecta
Duchenne dystrophy	Neuroleptic malignant syndrome
King syndrome	Myotonia congenita

however, it has not always been effective. In our laboratory, five out of six NMS patients exhibited abnormal halothane contractures (85), but we know of no reports of MH patients who also had NMS, or vice versa.

On occasion, NMS patients require electroconvulsive therapy under general anesthesia. Succinylcholine should be avoided in these patients and, if necessary, medium-acting nondepolarizing muscle relaxants, such as atracurium and vecuronium, should be used instead.

D. Sudden Infant Death Syndrome

Denborough has reported MH susceptibility (as determined by halothane contracture test) in 5 members of 15 families with SIDS cases (101). In contrast, Ellis and Halsall (18) found no increase in the incidence of MH in SIDS families. The relation between SIDS and MH remains inconclusive.

REFERENCES

1. Moschowitz AV: Postoperative heat stroke. *Surg Gynecol Obstet 23*:443–451, 1916.
2. Denborough MA, Lovell RRH: Anaesthetic deaths in a family. *Lancet 2*:45, 1960.
3. Denborough MA, Forster JFA, Lovell RH, et al.: Anesthetic deaths in a family. *Br J Anaesth 34*:395–396, 1962.
4. Britt BA, Locher WG, Kalow W: Hereditary aspects of malignant hyperthermia. *Can Anaesth Soc J 16*:89–98, 1969.
5. Britt BA, Kalow W, Gordon A, Humphrey JG, Newcastle NB: Malignant hyperthermia: An investigation of five patients. *Can Anaesth Soc J 20*:431–467, 1973.
6. Nelson TE, Jones EW, Hendrickson RL, et al.: Porcine malignant hyperthermia: Observations on the occurrence of pale, soft, exudative musculature among susceptible pigs. *Am J Vet Res 35*:347–350, 1974.
7. Campion DR, Topel DG: A review of the role of swine muscle in malignant hyperthermia. *J Anim Sci 41*:779–786, 1975.

8. Kalow W, Britt BA, Terreau ME, Haist C: Metabolic error of muscle metabolism after recovery from malignant hyperthermia. *Lancet 2*:895-898, 1970.
9. Britt BA: Malignant hyperthermia: A review, in *Handbook of Pharmacology*, Vol. 60 (Milton, AS, ed.), Springer-Verlag, Berlin, pp. 547-615, 1982.
10. Ording H: Incidence of malignant hyperthermia in Denmark. *Anesth Analg 64*:700-704, 1985.
11. Pan TH, Wollack AR, DeMarco JA: Malignant hyperthermia associated with enflurane: A case report. *Anesth Analg 54*: 47-49, 1975.
12. Cain PA, Ellis FR: Anesthesia for patients susceptible to malignant hyperpyrexia. *Br J Anaesth 49*:941, 1977.
13. Gronert GA: Malignant hyperthermia. *Anesthesiology 53*: 395-423, 1980.
14. Lunn JN, Farrow SC, Fowkes FGR, et al.: Epidemiology in anesthesia. *Br J Anaesth 59*:803-809, 1982.
15. Schwartz L, Rockoff MA, Koka BV: Masseter spasm with anesthesia: Incidence and implications. *Anesthesiology 61*: 772-775, 1984.
16. Rosenberg H, Reed S: In vitro contracture tests for susceptibility to malignant hyperthermia. *Anesth Analg 62*:415-420, 1983.
17. McPherson EW, Taylor CA: The King syndrome: Malignant hyperthermia, myopathy, and multiple anomalies. *Am J Med Genet 8*:159-165, 1981.
18. Ellis FR, Heffron JJA: Clinical and biochemical aspects of malignant hyperpyrexia, in *Recent Advances in Anaesthesia and Analgesia* (Atkinson RS, Adams AP, eds.), Churchill Livingstone, Edinburgh, pp. 173-207, 1985.
19. Eikelenboom G, Minkema D, Van Eldik P, Sybesma W: Inheritance of the malignant hyperthermia syndrome in Dutch Landrace swine, in *Malignant Hyperthermia* (Aldrete JA, Britt BA, eds.), Grune and Stratton, New York, pp. 141-146, 1978.
20. Moulds RFW, Denborough MA: Identification of susceptibility to malignant hyperpyrexia. *Br J Med 4*:245-247, 1974.
21. Ellis FR, Harriman DGF, Keaney NP, Kyei-Mensah K, Tyrrell JH: Halothane-induced muscle contracture as a cause of hyperpyrexia. *Br J Anaesth 43*:721-722, 1971.

22. Williams CH: The development of an animal model for the fulminant hyperthermia porcine stress syndrome, in *Malignant Hyperthermia: Current Concepts* (Henschel EO, ed.), Appleton-Century-Crofts, New York, pp. 117–140, 1977.
23. Williams CH, Lasley JF: The mode of inheritance of the fulminant hyperthermia stress syndrome in swine, in *Malignant Hyperthermia: Current Concepts* (Henschel EO, ed.), Appleton-Century-Crofts, New York, pp. 141–148, 1977.
24. Denborough MA: The pathopharmacology of malignant hyperpyrexia. *Pharmacol Ther 9*:357–365, 1980.
25. Cheah KS, Cheah AM: Membrane permeability in porcine malignant hyperthermia, in *Membrane Fluidity* (Kates M, Manson LA, eds.), Plenum, New York, pp. 661–687, 1984.
26. Harrison GG: Anaesthetic-induced malignant hyperpyrexia: A suggested method of treatment. *Br Med J 3*:454–456, 1971.
27. Hall GM, Lucke JN, Lister D: Porcine malignant hyperthermia IV: Neuromuscular blockade. *Br J Anaesth 48*: 1135–1141, 1976.
28. Britt BA, Endrenyi L, Frodis W, Scott E, Kalow, W: Comparison of effects of several inhalation anaesthetics on caffeine-induced contractures of normal and malignant hyperthermic skeletal muscle. *Can Anaesth Soc J 27*:12–15, 1980.
29. Nelson TE, Flewellen EH, Gloyna DF: Spectrum of susceptibility to malignant hyperthermia—Diagnostic dilemma. *Anesth Analg 62*:545–552, 1983.
30. Kalow W, Britt BA, Richter A: The caffeine test of isolated human muscle in relation to malignant hyperthermia. *Can Anaesth Soc J 24*:678–694, 1977.
31. Rosenberg H: International workshop on malignant hyperpyrexia. *Anesthesiology 54*:530–531, 1981.
32. Crocker BD, Okumura F, McCuaig DI, Denborough MA: Temperature monitoring during general anesthesia. *Br J Anaesth 52*:1223–1229, 1980.
33. Williams C: Some observations on the etiology of the fulminant hyperthermia-stress syndrome. *Prospect Biol Med 20*:120–130, 1976.

34. Gronert GA, Milde JH, Theye RA: Role of sympathetic activity in porcine malignant hyperthermia. *Anesthesiology 47*:411-415, 1977.
35. Campbell IT, Ellis FR, Evans RT, Mortimer MG: Studies of body temperatures, blood lactate, cortisol and free fatty acid levels during exercise in human subjects susceptible to malignant hyperpyrexia. *Acta Anaesthesiol Scand 27*:349-355, 1983.
36. Gronert GA, Heffron JJA, Milde JH, Theye RA: Porcine malignant hyperthermia: Role of skeletal muscle in increased oxygen consumption. *Can Anaesth Soc J 24*:130-109, 1977.
37. Tammisto T, Airaksinen M: Increase of creatine kinase activity in serum as a sign of muscular injury caused by intermittently administered suxamethonium during halothane anaesthesia. *Br J Anaesth 38*:510-515, 1966.
38. Innes RKR, Stromme JH: Rise in serum creatine phosphokinase associated with agents used in anaesthesia. *Br J Anaesth 45*:185-190, 1973.
39. Harrington JF, Ford DJ, Striker TW: Myoglobinemia after succinylcholine in children undergoing halothane and non-halothane anesthesia. *Anesthesiology 61*:A431, 1984.
40. Fletcher JE, Rosenberg H: In vitro interaction between halothane and succinylcholine in human skeletal muscle: Implications for malignant hyperthermia and masseter muscle rigidity. *Anesthesiology 63*:190-194, 1985.
41. Britt BA: Etiology and pathophysiology of malignant hyperthermia. *Fed Proc 38*:44-48, 1979.
42. Bennett D, Cain PA, Ellis FR, Louis CF, Stanton M: Calcium and magnesium contents of malignant hyperpyrexia-susceptible human muscle. *Br J Anaesth 49*:979-982, 1977.
43. Britt BA, Endrenyi L, Barclay RL, Cadman DL: Total Calcium content of skeletal muscle isolated from humans and pigs susceptible to malignant hyperthermia. *Br J Anaesth 47*:647-649, 1975.
44. Stadhouders AM, Viering WAL, Verburg MP, Ruitenbeek W, Sengers RCA: In vivo induced malignant hyperthermia in pigs. III. Localization of calcium in skeletal muscle mitochondria by means of electronmicroscopy and microprobe analysis. *Acta Anaesth Scand 28*:14-26, 1984.

45. Van den Hende C, Lister D, Muylle E, et al.: Malignant hyperthermia in Belgian Landrace pigs rested or exercised before exposure to halothane. *Br J Anaesth 48*:821–829, 1976.
46. Lewandowski KB: Rhabdomyolysis, myoglobinuria and hyperpyrexia caused by suxamethonium in a child with increased serum creatine kinase concentrations. *Br J Anaesth 53*:981–984, 1981.
47. Eng GD, Epstein BS, Engel WK, et al.: Malignant hyperthermia and central core disease in a child with congenital dislocating hips. *Arch Neurol 35*:189–197, 1978.
48. Stevens JNJ: A case of thyrotoxic crisis that mimicked malignant hyperthermia. *Anesthesiology 59*:263, 1983.
49. Gronert GA: Controversies in malignant hyperthermia. *Anesthesiology 59*:273–274, 1983.
50. Ording H, Ranklev E, Fletcher R: Investigation of malignant hyperthermia in Denmark and Sweden. *Br J Anaesth 56*: 1183–1190, 1984.
51. Blanck TJJ, Fischer YI, Thompson M, Muldoon S: Low molecular weight proteins in human malignant hyperthermia muscle. *Anesthesiology 61*:589–592, 1984.
52. Fletcher JE, Rosenberg, H, Hilf M: Electrophoresis of soluble muscle protein from human malignant hyperthermia susceptibles. *Anesthesiology 61*:A279, 1984.
53. Fletcher JE, Rosenberg H: Low molecular weight proteins in human malignant hyperthermia muscle (letter). *Anesthesiology 62*:849–850, 1985.
54. Sullivan JS, Denborough MA: The isolation and chemical characterization of skeletal muscle microsomes from swine susceptible to malignant hyperpyrexia. *Int J Biochem 14*: 741–745, 1982.
55. White MD, Collins JG, Denborough MA: The effect of dantrolene on skeletal muscle sarcoplasmic-reticulum function in malignant hyperpyrexia in pigs. *Biochem J 212*: 399–405, 1983.
56. Marjanen LA, Collins SP, Denborough MA: Calmodulin and malignant hyperpyrexia. *Biochem Med 32*:283–287, 1984.
57. Eng GD, Becker MJ, Muldoon SM: Electrodiagnostic tests in the detection of malignant hyperthermia. *Muscle Nerve 7*: 618–625, 1984.

58. Britt BA: Dantrolene. *Can Anaesth Soc J 31*:61–75, 1984.
59. Kolb ME, Horne ML, Martz R: Dantrolene in human malignant hyperthermia. *Anesthesiology 56*:254–262, 1982.
60. Martonosi AN: Mechanisms of Ca^{2+} release from sarcoplasmic reticulum of skeletal muscle. *Physiol Rev 64*:1240–1320, 1984.
61. Lopez JR, Alamo L, Jones D, Allen PD, Papp L, Gergely J, Streter FA: Dantrolene reverses the syndrome of malignant hyperthermia by reducing the level intracellular Ca^{2+} concentration. *Biophys J 47*:313a, 1985.
62. Austin KL, Denborough MA: Drug treatment of malignant hyperpyrexia. *Anaesth Intensive Care 5*:207–213, 1977.
63. Flewellen EH, Nelson TE: Intravenous dantrolene pharmacokinetics in malignant hyperthermia suspect patients. *Anesthesiology 63*:A300, 1985.
64. Flewellen EH, Nelson TE, Jones WP, Arens JF, et al.: Dantrolene dose response in awake man: Implications for management of malignant hyperthermia. *Anesthesiology 59*:275–280, 1983.
65. Zukaitis MG, Hoech GP, Williams CH, Simpson S: Verapamil attenuation of the malignant hyperthermia syndrome. *Anesthesiology 57*:A228, 1982.
66. Iwatsuki N, Koga Y, Amaha K: Calcium channel blocker for treatment of malignant hyperthermia. *Anesth Analg 62*:855–862, 1983.
67. Williams CH, Dozier SE, Ilias WK, Fulfer RT, Zukaitis MG, Noech GP: Treatment of malignant hyperthermia (MH) with diltiazem. *Fed Proc 44*:1638, 1985.
68. Saltzman LS, Kates RA, Corke BC, Norfleet EA, Heath KR: Hyperkalemia and cardiovascular collapse after verapamil and dantrolene administration in swine. *Anesth Analg 63*:473–478, 1984.
69. McGrath CJ, Lee JC, Rempel WE: Noneffectiveness of verapamil in preventing halothane-induced malignant hyperthermia in susceptible swine. *Am J Vet Res 45*:935–937, 1984.
70. Gallant EM, Foldes FF, Rempel WE, Gronert GA: Verapamil is not a therapeutic adjunct to dantrolene in porcine malignant hyperthermia. *Anesth Analg 64*:601–606, 1985.

71. Verburg MP, Oerlemans FT, Van Bennekom CA, et al.: In vivo induced malignant hyperthermia in pigs: I. Physiological and biochemical changes and the influence of dantrolene sodium. *Acta Anaesth Scand 28*:1-8, 1984.
72. Denborough MA, Hudson MC, Foster JFA, et al.: Biochemical changes in malignant hyperthermia. *Lancet 1*:1137-1138, 1975.
73. Hall GM, Lucke JN, Lowell R, Lister D: Porcine malignant hyperthermia VII: Hepatic metabolism. *Br J Anaesth 52*: 11-17, 1980.
74. Larach MG, Rosenberg H: Evaluation and management of pediatric patients for diagnostic muscle biopsy for malignant hyperthermia susceptibility. *Anesthesiology 59*:A228, 1983.
75. Nelson TE, Bedell DM, Jones EW: Porcine malignant hyperthermia: Effects of temperature and extracellular calcium concentration on halothane-induced contracture of susceptible skeletal muscle. *Anesthesiology 42*:301-306, 1975.
76. Vaughan MS, Cork C, Vaughan RW: Inaccuracy of liquid crystal thermometry to identify core temperature trends in postoperative adults. *Anesth Analg 61*:284-287, 1982.
77. Berkowitz A, Rosenberg H: Femoral block with mepivecaine for muscle biopsy in malignant hyperthermia patients. *Anesthesiology 62*:651-652, 1985.
78. Fletcher JE, Rosenberg H, Hilf M: Effects of midazolam on directly stimulated muscle biopsies from control and malignant hyperthermia positive patients. *Can Anaesth Soc J 31*: 377-381, 1984.
79. Ruhland GA, Hinkle A: Malignant hyperthermia after oral and intravenous pretreatment with dantrolene in a patient susceptible to malignant hyperthermia. *Anesthesiology 60*: 159-160, 1984.
80. Reed SB, Strobel GE: An in vitro model of malignant hyperthermia. *Anesthesiology 48*:254-259, 1978.
81. Gronert GA, Milde JH: Variations in onset of porcine malignant hyperthermia. *Anesth Analg 60*:499-503, 1981.
82. Skarpa M, Doyan AD, Follenfant M, et a.: Toxicity testing of atracurium. *Br J Anaesth 55*:S27-29, 1983.
83. Buzello W, Williams CH, Chandria P, et al.: Vecuronium and porcine malignant hyperthermia. *Anesth Analg 64*:515-519, 1985.

84. Caroff SN: The neuroleptic malignant syndrome. *J Clin Psychiatry 41*:79–83, 1980.
85. Caroff S, Rosenberg H, Gerber JC: Neuroleptic malignant syndrome and malignant hyperthermia. *Lancet 1*:244, 1983.
86. Rosenberg H: Malignant hyperthermia syndrome. *Anesth Analg 56*:466, 1977.
87. Noble WH, McKee D, Gates B: Malignant hyperthermia with rigidity successfully treated with procainamide. *Anesthesiology 39*:450–451, 1973.
88. Gronert GA, Milde JH, Theye RA: Porcine malignant hyperthermia induced by halothane and succinylcholine: Failure of treatment with procaine or procainamide. *Anesthesiology 44*: 124–132, 1976.
89. Moulds RFW, Denborough MA: Procaine in malignant hyperpyrexia. *Br Med J 4*:526–528, 1972.
90. Strobel GE, Bianchi CP: An in-vitro model of anesthetic hypertonic hyperpyrexia, halothane-caffeine-induced muscle contractures: Prevention of contractures by procainamide. *Anesthesiology 35*:465–473, 1971.
91. Wingard DW, Bobko S: Failure of lidocaine to trigger porcine malignant hyperthermia. *Anesth Analg 58*:99–103, 1979.
92. Harison GG, Morrell DF: Response of MHS swine to IV infusion of lidocaine and bupivecaine. *Br J Anaesth 52*: 385–387, 1980.
93. Hall GM, Lucke JN, Lister D: Porcine malignant hyperthermia V: Fatal hyperthermia in the Pietrain pig, associated with the infusion of alpha adrenergic agonists. *Br J Anaesth 49*:855–863, 1977.
94. Morrison DH: Placental transfer of dantrolene (letter). *Anesthesiology 59*:265, 1983.
95. Neubauer K, Kaufman RD: Another use for mass spectrometry: Detection and monitoring of malignant hyperthermia. *Anesth Analg 64*:837–839, 1983.
96. Rosenberg H, Paterson TH: Duchenne's muscular dystrophy and malignant hyperthermia: Another warning (letter). *Anesthesiology 59*:362, 1983.
97. Mitchell MM, Ali HH, Savarese JJ: Myotonia and neuromuscular blocking agents. *Anesthesiology 49*:44–48, 1978.

98. Granato JE, Stern BJ, Ringel A: Neuroleptic malignant syndrome: Successful treatment with dantrolene and bromocriptine. *Ann Neurol 14*:89-90, 1983.
99. Goulon M, de Rohan-Chabot P, Elkharrat D, et al.: Beneficial effects of dantrolene in the treatment of neuroleptic malignant syndrome: A report of two cases. *Neurology 33*:516-518, 1983.
100. Coons DJ, Hillman FJ, Marshall RW: Treatment of neuroleptic malignant syndrome with dantrolene sodium: A case report. *Am J Psychiatry 139*:944-945, 1982.
101. Denborough MA, Galloway GJ, Hopkinson KC: Malignant hyperpyrexia and sudden infant death. *Lancet 2*:1068-1069, 1982.
102. Fletcher JE, Rosenberg H: In vitro muscle contractures induced by halothane and succinylcholine: II. Human skeletal muscle from normal and malignant hyperthermia susceptible patients. *Br J Anaesth*, in press.
103. Rosenberg H, Fletcher JE: Masseter muscle rigidity and malignant hyperthermia susceptibility. *Anesth Analg 65*: 161-164, 1986.
104. Lopez JR, Alamo L, Caputo C, Wikenski J, Ledezma D: Intracellular ionized calcium concentrations in muscle from humans with malignant hyperthermia. *Muscle Nerve 8*:355-358, 1985.
105. Gronert GA, Ahern CP, Milde JH, White RD: Effect of CO_2, calcium, digoxin and potassium on cardiac and skeletal muscle metabolism in malignant hyperthermia susceptible swine. *Anesthesiology 64*:24-28, 1986.

6

Muscle Relaxants and the Patient with Renal and/or Hepatic Failure

STEPHEN M. RUPP
University of California, San Francisco, San Francisco, California

I. INTRODUCTION

Clinicians who care for the critically ill are frequently faced with patients who have renal or hepatic failure. Often these patients have complicated illnesses which involve multiple organ failure. When these patients undergo surgery or during mechanical ventilation in an intensive care unit, they may receive nondepolarizing muscle relaxants. Because the kidney and liver are major routes of elimination for most drugs, renal and hepatic diseases may alter the elimination of nondepolarizing muscle relaxants. Moreover, changes in hydration, protein binding, and acid-base status may alter the distribution of these drugs. The response of the neuromuscular junction to muscle relaxants may also be altered.

The purpose of this chapter is to review the pharmacokinetics and pharmacodynamics of nondepolarizing muscle relaxants in normal individuals and then to assess the changes that occur in renal and hepatic failures. Antagonists of nondepolarizing muscular blockade will also be discussed. Through this, we hope to guide the clinician to a rational choice and use of these drugs.

The reader may ask, "Why pharmacokinetics and pharmacodynamics?" The term pharmacodynamics describes the effect a drug has on the body. In this context, it relates to the onset of paralysis, intensity of neuromuscular blockade, sensitivity of the neuromuscular junction to muscle relaxants, duration of paralysis, and rate of recovery. The term pharmacokinetics describes the manner in which the drug is distributed, metabolized, and excreted by the body. The changes in the pharmacodynamics of nondepolarizing muscle relaxants in illness are reflections of altered pharmacokinetics. Simply stated, the effect of these relaxants can be related to the concentration of the drug in the blood. Numerous studies have demonstrated this relationship (1-5).

Detailed explanations and derivations of pharmacokinetic principles are beyond the scope of this book. Readers unfamiliar with these concepts are referred to excellent reviews (6-8) and textbooks (9-11). In this chapter, we will consider the volume of distribution during the elimination phase (Vd_β) and at steady-state (Vdss), the clearance (Cl, the volume of blood from which the drug is completely cleared per unit time), and elimination half-life ($t_{1/2}\beta$, the time necessary for the drug concentration to decline by one-half during the elimination phase). Discussion of the volume of the central compartment (V_1, representing the blood volume and rapidly equilibrating tissues) and of the distribution half-life ($t_{1/2}\alpha$) will be limited because these parameters are minimally affected by renal and hepatic disease.

There is no uniform method of assessment of the sensitivity of the neuromuscular junction to muscle relaxants. Different researchers use different methods and therefore the results are inconsistent. In general, sensitivity is expressed as the plasma concentration at a certain degree of neuromuscular blockade (e.g., 50%) either during the recovery phase (e.g., Cp_{50}) or at steady state (e.g., $Cpss_{50}$).

Six nondepolarizing muscle relaxants currently available in the United States will be discussed in this chapter: atracurium, d-tubocurarine, gallamine, metocurine, pancuronium, and vecuronium.

II. PHARMACOKINETICS OF NONDEPOLARIZING MUSCLE RELAXANTS IN NORMAL SUBJECTS

A. Distribution

The nondepolarizing muscle relaxants share many physicochemical properties and therefore they have similar diffusion and distribution characteristics. Their molecules are large (molecular weight 600-1000) and they contain one, two, or three quaternary ammonium groups (Fig. 1). The molecules are positively charged at physiological pH and tend to be highly ionized at any pH because of the quaternary ammonium groups. Because of their high ionization, the molecules of nondepolarizing muscle relaxants are water soluble and therefore they hardly cross lipoid membrane. They are largely confined to the extracellular space.

B. Protein Binding

Plasma and tissue protein binding may have a profound effect on the volume of distribution and disposition of drugs. The free or unbound fraction of a drug is the only portion available for pharmacological action at receptor sites. Similarly, it is the only portion of a drug available for metabolism and excretion. The larger the unbound fraction, the more free drug is available for distribution to areas outside the plasma volume. Familiarity with the degree of protein binding in health and disease helps in understanding the pharmacokinetics of drugs.

Unfortunately, there is no clear consensus on the extent of protein binding by nondepolarizing muscle relaxants. Several laboratory techniques have been used to determine protein binding of muscle relaxants: Equilibrium dialysis (12-15), gel filtration (12), electrophoresis (16), and butyrylcholinesterase inhibition (17). However, the results vary widely. In general, protein binding of these drugs is low (<90%) and sensitive to changes in temperature and pH. This is apparently the reason for the inconsistent reports on protein binding by muscle relaxants. This author believes that equilibrium dialysis is the best method for determining protein binding of nondepolarizing muscle relaxants in vivo (15,18).

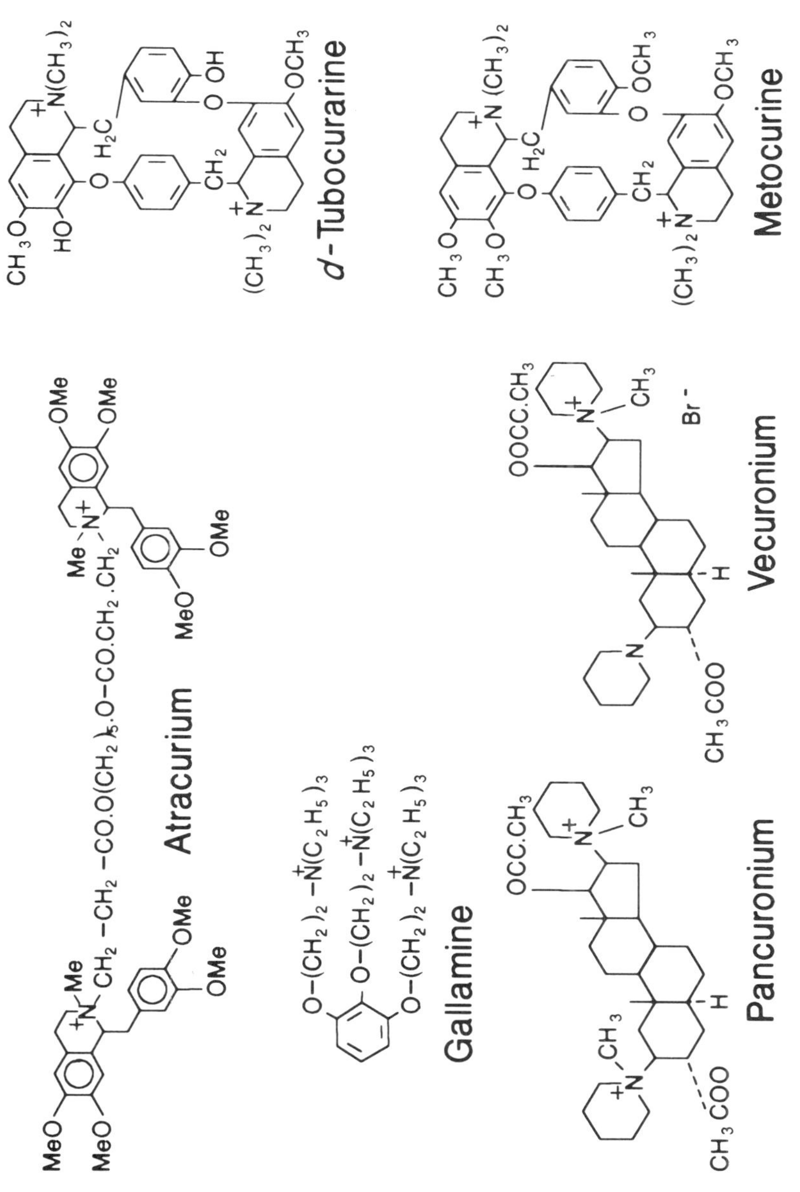

Figure 1 Chemical structures of the six nondepolarizing muscle relaxants available in the United States. All are large molecules, with one, two, or three quaternary ammonium groups and are ionized at physiological pH.

Table 1 Normal Values of Protein Binding and Pharmacokinetic Parameters

Drug (Refs.)	Protein binding (%)	Vdss (L/kg)	Elimination half-life (hr)
d-Tubocurarine (11,12,14,19,20,99)	40-56	0.3-0.5	2-5.8
Metocurine (14,20,21,27)	35-70	0.42-0.57	3.6-5.8
Pancuronium (13,25,33,34,46,55,100)	10-20	0.14-0.38	1.7-2.4
Gallamine (22,38,101)	16	0.21	2.2±0.6
Vecuronium (5,30,37,47,48,51)	24-30	0.18-0.26	0.5-1.3
Atracurium (17,49,50)	82	0.18	0.33

Table 1 lists the muscle relaxants and their percent of plasma protein binding as determined by equilibrium dialysis. Of all muscle relaxants, d-tubocurarine is the most highly protein bound (40-50%) (12,14,19,20). It apparently binds albumin, o_1 acid glycoprotein, and gamma globulin (14,15). The binding of metocurine is similar to that of d-tubocurarine, but the reported range of values is wider (35-70%) (20,21). Gallamine (16%) (22), pancuronium (10-29%) (5,13), and vecuronium (24-30%) (5) bind proteins to a lesser degree.

Because nondepolarizing muscle relaxants have low plasma protein binding capacity, disease-induced changes in plasma protein concentration have minimal effect on their pharmacological effect.

Tissue binding (especially to cartilage and connective tissue) appears to play an important role in the distribution (23-25) and "nonrecoverable" elimination (26) of metocurine and d-tubocurarine. Chagas (24) demonstrated that acid mucopolysaccharides can bind large quantities of metocurine. Similarly, Olsen et al. (23) showed extensive binding of d-tubocurarine and

Clearance (ml/kg min)	% Metabolized	% Renal excretion	% Hepatic excretion
1-2.7	Very low	46-95% in 48 hr	12% (6-18%) in 48 hr
1.2-1.8	Very low	46-58% in 48 hr	2.1% in 48 hr
1.0-2.0	25% to 3-OH Pancuronium <5% 17-OH Pancuronium 3,17-OH Pancuronium	25% as 3-OH 5% as 17- or 3,17-OH 67% total	11%
1.2	0	95% in 24-30 hr	0.1-0.4%
3	<30% 5%-3-OH Vecuronium	10-30%	46%
5.1-6.1	100%		

metocurine to the chondroitin sulfate in cartilage. Brotherton and Matteo (27) estimated that 50–75% of a metocurine dose may be bound in this manner. Because of tissue binding, the calculated volume of distribution of d-tubocurarine and metocurine exceeds the actual volume of extracellular fluid (20,27,28). Tissue binding also explains why d-tubocurarine and metocurine have greater volumes of distribution at steady state (Vdss) than other nondepolarizing muscle relaxants (Table 1). The degree of tissue binding of pancuronium, vecuronium, gallamine, and atracurium is unknown.

Hepatic uptake and storage of steroidal nondepolarizing muscle relaxants (pancuronium and especially vecuronium) represent another aspect of drug distribution (29,30). In cats, 3 min after the administration of Org 6368 (a derivative of pancuronium), 40% of the dose was taken up by the liver (29). Based on liver biopsy analysis, Bencini (30) estimated that 40–80% of an intravenous dose of vecuronium may be taken up by the liver within 30 min after its administration. The large hepatic uptake of vecuronium may be the cause of its short duration of action.

C. Metabolism

The degree of metabolism that nondepolarizing muscle relaxants undergo varies widely, ranging from less than 2% for gallamine to potentially 100% for atracurium (Table 1). Atracurium was designed by Stenlake et al. (31) to undergo a nonenzymatic pH and temperature-dependent spontaneous degradation (Hofmann elimination). In vivo, however, in addition to the nonenzymatic degradation, an enzymatic ester hydrolysis also occurs. The byproducts of atracurium metabolism have no neuromuscular-blocking effect, and they are excreted by the liver and the kidney (32).

Hepatic biodegradation has been demonstrated for pancuronium (33,34) and vecuronium (35). A small fraction (20–30%) of pancuronium undergoes metabolism as follows: Single deacetylation to 3-hydroxypancuronium (up to 25%) and to 17-hydroxypancuronium (<5%), and double deacetylation to 3,17-dihydroxypancuronium (<5%) (33,36). The rest is excreted as the parent compound.

The metabolism of vecuronium is also limited (35,37). Spontaneous deacetylation occurs in the liver and the byproducts are 3-hydroxy and 17-hydroxy derivatives. The 3-OH metabolites of both vecuronium and pancuronium are roughly one-half as potent at the neuromuscular junction as the parent compounds. The 17-OH and 3,17-OH metabolites are far less active (34,37).

The metabolism of metocurine and d-tubocurarine in the liver appears to be less than 5% (20). Gallamine does not appear to be metabolized at all (38) (Table 1).

D. Elimination

Pharmacokinetic studies have identified four routes of elimination of nondepolarizing muscle relaxants: Renal, hepatic, biotransformation (including Hofmann elimination), and nonrecoverable elimination (e.g., tissue binding). Biotransformation and nonrecoverable elimination were discussed above. In this section, we will examine normal renal and hepatic elimination mechanisms and then the individual elimination of each nondepolarizing muscle relaxant in order of decreasing dependence on renal excretion.

1. Renal Mechanisms

Assessment of renal excretion of a drug is typically done by collecting urine for a period of 24–48 hr after a drug was administered and measuring the amount of drug recovered. Nondepolarizing muscle relaxants are polar and filter freely through the glomerulus. The renal clearance of these drugs does not exceed the glomerular filtration rate (1–2 ml/kg/min), and therefore, there is little evidence of tubular secretion. Tubular reabsorption may possibly occur, but there are no data to support this statement.

Unlike nondepolarizing muscle relaxants, acetylcholinesterase inhibitors apparently undergo tubular secretion, in addition to glomerular filtration. Active secretion of neostigmine has been shown in animals (39). Renal clearance of the inhibitors ranges from 4 to 6 ml/kg/min.

2. Hepatic Mechanisms

Biliary excretion of d-tubocurarine has been studied in an isolated perfused rat liver (40,41). d-Tubocurarine diffuses passively into hepatocytes and is concentrated in lysosomes (42). The lysosomes empty their contents into biliary canaliculi. The bile to plasma concentration ratio for d-tubocurarine may be as high as 100 to 1 (41). An active transport system, dependent on a Na^+-K^+ activated ATPase, appears to be involved in the biliary elimination of d-tubocurarine (43). A rise in plasma level of bile acids, as seen in patients with cholestasis, inhibits the uptake of d-tubocurarine by the liver (41).

Westra et al. (44) showed that a rise in plasma level of bile salts potentiated the neuromuscular effect of pancuronium and vecuronium. They speculated that this was due to inhibition of hepatic uptake of these drugs.

Assessment of hepatic excretion in human subjects is difficult and requires collection of bile samples. Because of sampling errors (leakage of bile around the T tube) and because some of the drug is often excreted after the sampling has been completed, the cumulative recovery of a drug from urine and bile rarely approaches 100%. Typically, only 50–75% of the drug is accounted for.

3. Elimination Pathways for Specific Drugs

The kidney is the sole pathway for gallamine elimination (24,38,45). The amount excreted in 24 hr is highly variable (56-100%), and depends on the operative site (in abdominal and pelvic operations, the excretion is slower), the patient's age, and degree of surgical stress (38).

Metocurine is second only to gallamine in its dependence on renal excretion. Brotherton and Matteo (27) found that 43% of a metocurine dose was excreted by the kidneys in 24 hr. Meijer et al. (20) found that 46–58% was excreted in 48 hr. Only 2.1% of a metocurine dose was found unchanged in the bile (20). Since there is no evidence of metocurine metabolism (20), apparently the remaining metocurine is stored in the body and eventually it is excreted by the kidneys over a long period of time.

Within 24 hr after administration of pancuronium, Duvaldestin et al. (46) recovered 67% of the drug in the urine in the form of the parent compound and its metabolites. In other studies (33,36), about 25% of the injected pancuronium appeared in the urine in the form of 3-OH metabolite and less than 5% each in the form of the 17-OH and 3,17-dehydroxy metabolites. Approximately 11% of the pancuronium was excreted in the bile as the parent compound and its metabolites (33).

d-Tubocurarine is excreted unchanged: 46–95% in the urine and 6–18% in the bile within 48 hr (20). Thus, although the differences are small, d-tubocurarine appears to be less dependent on the kidney for elimination than either metocurine or pancuronium.

Of all the nondepolarizing muscle relaxants, vecuronium is the most dependent on biliary excretion. In rats, Upton et al. (47) recovered 46% of vecuronium in the bile within 7 hr. In humans, it is estimated that 40–50% of the drug is eliminated by the liver (30). The kidney excreted 10–30% within 12 hr, a third of which was in the form of the 3-OH metabolite (30).

Atracurium does not depend on the kidney or the liver for elimination because it is biodegraded by Hofmann elimination and ester hydrolysis. However, the parent compound and its metabolites are normally found in bile and urine (32).

E. Normal Pharmacokinetic Values

1. Nondepolarizing Muscle Relaxants

The normal pharmacokinetic values of nondepolarizing muscle relaxants are listed in Table 1. The volume of distribution at steady-state ranges from 0.14 L/kg to 0.57 L/kg. These values are rough approximations of the extracellular fluid volume. The volume of distribution for metocurine and d-tubocurarine are somewhat larger, probably because of tissue binding (see Sect. II.B). The clearance rates for d-tubocurarine, metocurine, pancuronium, and gallamine are in the range of 1-2 ml/kg/min, whereas the clearance rates of vecuronium and atracurium are 3 ml/kg/min (48) and 5.1-6.1 ml/kg/min (49,50), respectively. Because of their high rates of clearance, the elimination half-lives of vecuronium and atracurium are shorter than those of other muscle relaxants: 0.5-1.3 hr and 0.33 hr for vecuronium (51,48) and atracurium (50), respectively, versus 1.7-5.8 hr for the longer acting nondepolarizing muscle relaxants.

2. Acetylcholinesterase Inhibitors

Acetylcholinesterase inhibitors (edrophonium, neostigmine, pyridostigmine) are used to antagonize nondepolarizing muscle relaxants. Like muscle relaxants, they too are quaternary ammonium compounds, but their volume of distribution is approximately twice as large as that of muscle relaxants (Table 4). The degree of protein binding of inhibitors is unknown. Their clearance rate (8 ml/kg/min) is three- to fivefold greater than that of nondepolarizing muscle relaxants. By comparing clearance rates and elimination half-lives in patients with renal failure to those in normal subjects, it was determined that 50-75% of an inhibitor is excreted by the kidney. The rest is presumably eliminated by hepatic metabolism and excretion (51).

III. RENAL FAILURE

In 1971, Riordan and Gilbertson (52) reported a case of prolonged paralysis in a patient with renal failure following d-tubocurarine administration. They speculated that the cause was delayed renal

Table 2 Pharmacokinetics of Nondepolarizing Relaxants in for Elimination

Drug	Ref.	Patient group	N	Vdβ (L/kg)
Atracurium	50	Normal	10	0.182 ± 12
		Renal failure	9	0.224 ± 16
	57	Normal	6	0.159 ± 21
		Renal and hepatic failure	7	0.207 ± 49[a]
Vecuronium	48	Normal	4	—
		Renal failure	5	—
	30	Normal	5	—
		Renal failure	7	—
d-Tubocurarine	1	Normal	10	—
		Renal failure	10	—
Metocurine	27	Normal	5	0.472 ± 0.055
		Renal failure	5	0.353 ± 0.053[a]
Pancuronium	59	Normal	6	21 ± 3.4
		Renal failure	6	15 ± 6.0[a]
	55	Normal	6	0.148 ± .014
		Renal failure	7	0.236 ± .025[a]
	36	Normal	7	0.338 ± 0.074
		Renal failure	10	0.330 ± 0.201
Gallamine	56	Normal	17	0.225 ± 0.054
		Renal failure	8	0.290 ± 0.096[a]

[a]Significant difference from normal group, $p < 0.05$.

excretion of d-tubocurarine. This contradicted previous belief that recovery from d-tubocurarine in renal failure was normal (53). Others also reported prolonged paralysis (54) and "recurarization" (55) in patients with renal failure after pancuronium or d-tubocurarine administration. Since then, the pharmacokinetics of all the nondepolarizing muscle relaxants currently in use in the United States have been investigated.

Since renal elimination is the predominant route for gallamine (95%), metocurine (40–90%), pancuronium (67%), and d-tubocurarine (40–50%), renal failure has a major effect on the pharmacokinetics of these drugs. The pharmacokinetics of vecuronium (renal excretion 10–30%) and of atracurium (renal

Renal Failure in Order of Increasing Dependence on the Kidney

Vdss (L/kg)	Cl (ml/kg min)	$t_{1/2}\beta$ (hr)	Values
—	6.1 ± 0.3	0.34 ± 0.02	Mean ± SEM
—	6.7 ± 0.6	0.40 ± 0.02	
—	5.3 ± 0.8	0.35 ± 0.03	
—	6.5 ± 1.5	0.37 ± 0.07	Mean ± SD
0.194 ± 41	3.0 ± 0.3	1.33 ± 0.23	Mean ± SD
0.239 ± 63	2.5 ± 0.6	1.62 ± 0.63	
0.252	4.93 ± 0.8	1.6	Mean ± SD
0.423	2.6 ± .04[a]	2.5[a]	
0.25	1.4	1.4	
0.25	1.5[a]	2.2[a]	
—	1.2 ± 0.3	6.0 ± 0.95	Mean ± SEM
—	0.38 ± .06[a]	11.4 ± 1.5[a]	
—	—	4.1 ± 2.6	Mean ± SEM
—	—	17.5 ± 16.5[a]	
—	1.015 ± 0.110	1.67	Mean ± SEM
—	0.309 ± 0.030[a]	8.15[a]	
0.261 ± 0.046	1.8 ± 0.7	2.2 ± 0.42	Mean ± SEM
0.296 ± 0.158	0.88 ± 0.3[a]	4.3 ± 2.1[a]	
0.207 ± 0.048	1.2 ± 0.3	2.2	Mean ± SEM
0.285 ± 0.092[a]	0.24 ± .08[a]	12.5[a]	

excretion nearly 0%) are affected very little by renal failure. Table 2 summarizes the pharmacokinetics of muscle relaxants in patients with normal and abnormal renal function in an increasing order of dependence on renal excretion.

The volume of distribution of nondepolarizing muscle relaxants in patients with renal failure has been reported as increased (56-58), unchanged (1,30,48,50,59), or decreased (27,60). The discrepancies in these reports are probably due to the variable state of hydration of the patients in the above studies. For example, Brotherton and Matteo (27) studied the pharmacokinetics of metocurine in patients who were dialyzed until they reached "dry weight." Not surprisingly, they found a decreased volume of distribution (Table 2).

Changes in plasma protein levels in patients with renal failure probably have no significant effect on the volume of distribution of muscle relaxants because protein binding plays only a minor role in the pharmacokinetics of these drugs (12).

While the volume of distribution of muscle relaxants in renal failure varies, their clearance rates decrease consistently and are inversely related to the dependence of each individual muscle relaxant on renal excretion. The decrease in renal clearance results in prolonged elimination half-life and increased duration of action.

A. Atracurium

Since atracurium does not depend on the kidney for excretion, its elimination half-life and duration of action are not prolonged in patients with renal failure (50,58,61) (Table 2). Fahey et al. (50) found no change in the kinetics (Table 2) or duration of action and rate of recovery from atracurium in these patients (Table 3). Hunter et al. (61) also found no difference in duration of action. In a study of patients with both hepatic and renal failures, Ward and Neill (58) found no change in clearance or elimination half-life of atracurium. These studies suggest that atracurium is an excellent choice for patients with impaired or with no renal function.

Laudanosine, a major metabolite of atracurium, accumulates in patients with renal failure, and its serum level remains elevated for a prolonged period of time (62). In large doses, laudanosine has been shown to cause central nervous system stimulation in dogs (63) and rabbits (64). It also increases the minimum alveolar concentration (MAC) of halothane in rabbits (65), and in dogs it causes electroencephalographic changes of arousal during halothane anesthesia (66). The clinical importance of laudanosine in patients with renal failure, particularly following repeated doses of atracurium, has not been determined.

B. Vecuronium

Vecuronium is only slightly dependent on renal elimination (10–30%), and therefore, its elimination should be minimally affected by renal failure. Indeed, Fahey et al. (48) found no

Table 3 Pharmacodynamics of Atracurium and Vecuronium in Renal Failure

Drug	Ref.	Patient group	N	Dose (mg/kg)	Onset (min)	Duration (min)	Recovery (min)[d]
Atracurium	50	Normal	10	0.5	1.8 ± 0.1	70 ± 5[a]	11 ± 1
		Renal failure	10	0.5	2.0 ± 0.4	77 ± 3[a]	13 ± 3
	60	Normal	25	0.5		39 ± 10[b]	
		Renal failure	21	0.5		35 ± 11[b]	
Vecuronium	48	Normal	4	0.14	2.1 ± 0.6	104 ± 13[c]	21 ± 3
		Renal failure	4	0.14	1.8 ± 0.7	104 ± 46[c]	29 ± 23

[a]Duration: Time from injection to 95% recovery of control twitch tension (MEAN ± SEM).
[b]Duration: Time from injection to 10% recovery of control twitch tension (MEAN ± SEM).
[c]Duration: Time from injection to 90% recovery of control twitch tension (MEAN ± S.D.).
[d]Recovery: Time from 25% to 75% of control twitch tension during recovery phase.

changes in volume of distribution, clearance, elimination half-life, or recovery time from vecuronium in these patients (Tables 2 and 3). In contrast, Bencini et al. (30) found a 50% decrease in clearance, an increase in volume of distribution, and a 50% increase in elimination half-life. The duration of action was not reported. More studies are necessary to determine the exact effect of renal failure on the pharmacokinetics of vecuronium. At this time, it seems appropriate to conclude that although the elimination of vecuronium is affected by renal failure, elimination of gallamine, pancuronium, metocurine, and d-tubocurarine is affected significantly more.

C. d-Tubocurarine

The clearance of d-tubocurarine is reduced and its elimination half-life is increased in renal failure (1) (Fig. 2; Table 2). Normally, 40–50% of the parent compound is excreted by the kidney and 12% in the bile (20) (Table 1). However, in animals in renal failure (achieved by ligation of the renal pedicles), the biliary excretion of d-tubocurarine is increased up to 39% (67). This is why d-tubocurarine was favored over gallamine, pancuronium, and metocurine prior to the introduction of atracurium and vecuronium.

d-Tubocurarine has been implicated as causing prolonged paralysis (52,54,68) and recurarization (55) in anephric patients. Others have reported normal duration of action in these patients (52). Gibaldi et al. (26), using pharmacokinetic modeling to reconcile these contradictory reports, showed that when a patient in renal failure is given a small dose of d-tubocurarine, the plasma concentration of this drug declines at a normal rate, primarily because of redistribution and nonrecoverable elimination (deposition in tissues). However, when large or repeated doses of d-tubocurarine are given, the kidney assumes a major role in the elimination of this drug. In the presence of renal failure, therefore, the plasma concentration of d-tubocurarine following large doses of this drug remains elevated for a long period of time.

D. Pancuronium

Two-thirds of a pancuronium dose is normally eliminated by the kidney (46), and therefore, if given in renal failure, prolonged

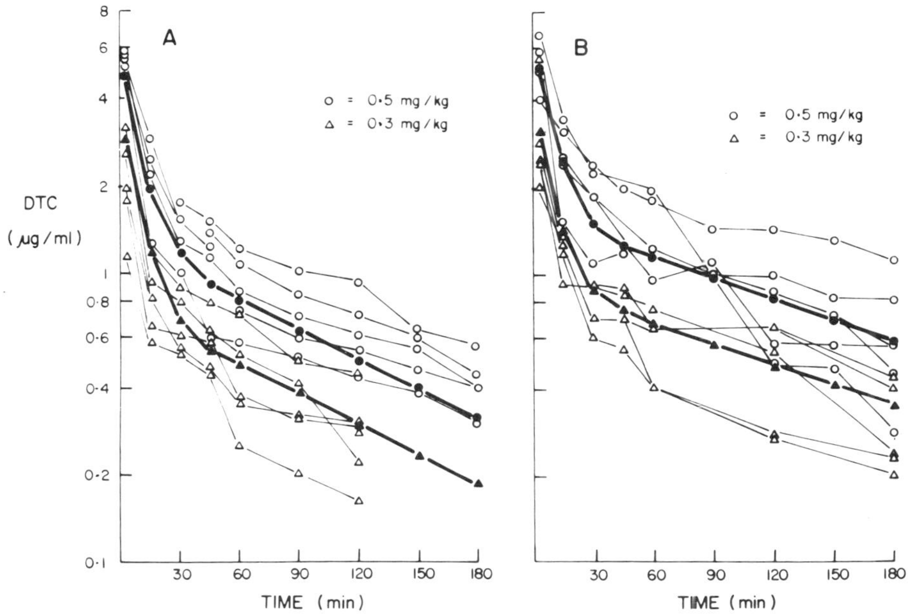

Figure 2 Plasma concentration of d-tubocurarine versus time relationships for normal patients (A) and patients with renal failure (B). The solid dark line represents the estimated mean population response for the dose and type of patient. The fall in plasma concentration of d-tubocurarine is delayed in patients with renal failure. (From Ref. 1, used with permission.)

paralysis may occur (36,38). Similarly to d-tubocurarine, pancuronium has been implicated in recurarization (55), and according to two reports, hemodialysis was necessary to reverse its neuromuscular blockade in patients with renal failure (69,70). The clearance of pancuronium is reduced by one-half to two-thirds, whereas the volume of distribution is only minimally affected (Table 2).

Although pancuronium is metabolized up to 25% (33,34), the metabolites accumulate in renal failure because they normally depend on renal excretion. The metabolites, especially 3-hydroxypancuronium, have some neuromuscular-blocking activity (34) and they further prolong paralysis. This results in a two- to fourfold increase in elimination half-life (36,56,60).

E. Metocurine

Metocurine clearance is reduced by two-thirds in renal failure, whereas its volume of distribution is decreased by one-third (27). This results in a twofold increase in elimination half-life (from 6 to 11 hr; Table 2). The investigators also found that patients with renal failure were resistant to metocurine. There are no other reports of altered sensitivity to metocurine or to any other muscle relaxant in renal failure.

Since only 2% of metocurine is normally eliminated in the bile, hepatic elimination can not compensate for a decrease in renal excretion of this drug. In view of this, there is little reason to use metocurine in patients with renal failure.

F. Gallamine

Gallamine-induced prolonged paralysis in patients with renal failure has been reported several times (71–75). This is not surprising since gallamine is virtually 100% eliminated by the kidney (24,38,45). Ramzan et al. (57) found an increase in elimination half-life from 2.2 to 12.5 hr in patients with renal failure (Table 2). Nevertheless, one clinical report demonstrated spontaneous recovery from small doses of gallamine (76), probably due to redistribution and tissue uptake of the drug (77). In view of the availability of alternative drugs, this author sees no reason to use gallamine in patients with renal failure.

G. Antagonists of Neuromuscular Blockade

For many years recurarization in renal failure was felt to be due to "wearing off" of the effects of the acetylcholinesterase inhibitor before the muscle relaxant was completely eliminated. This concept has been refuted by pharmacokinetic studies conducted by Cronnelly et al. (78,79) and Morris et al. (80,81) (Table 4; Fig. 3). In general, the clearance of acetylcholinesterase inhibitors

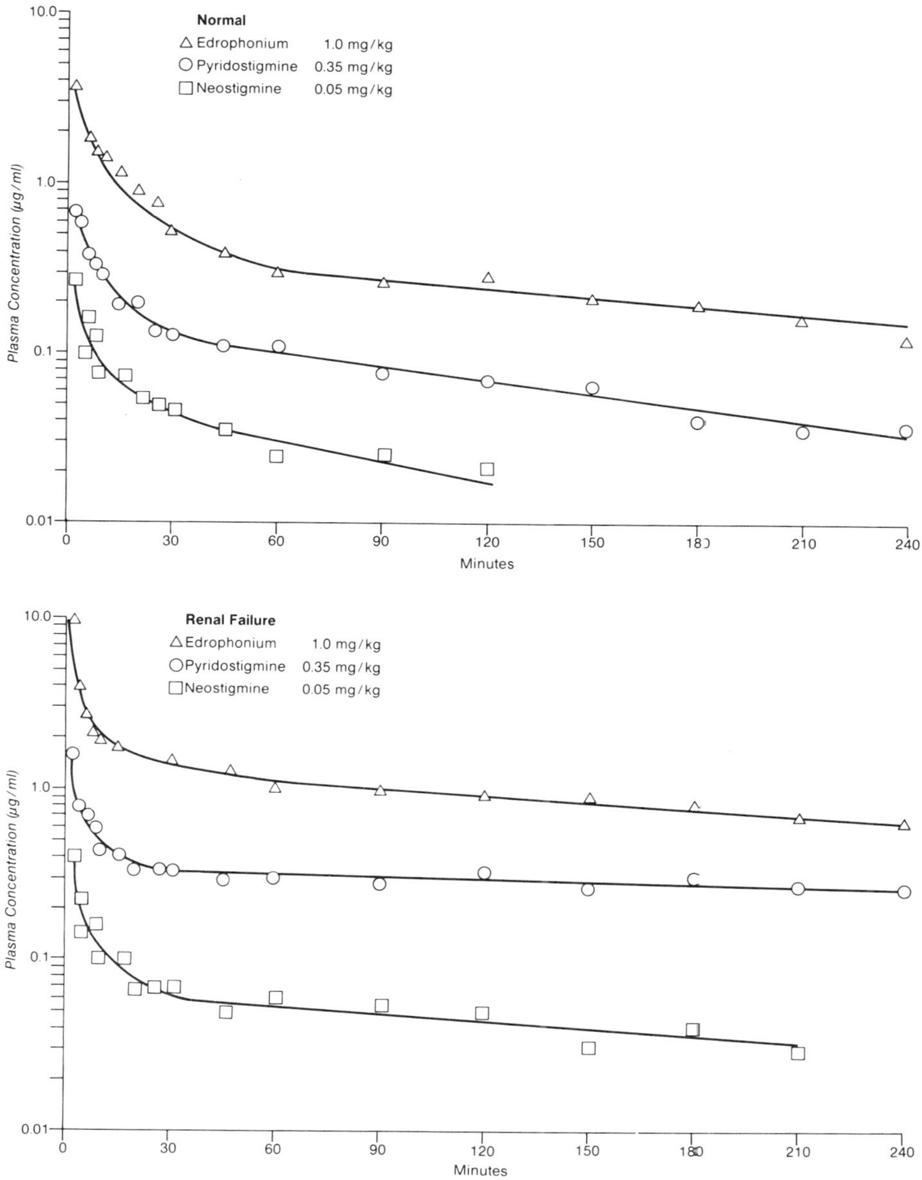

Figure 3 Plasma concentration of the acetylcholinesterase inhibitors versus time in normal patients and patients with renal failure. The fall in plasma concentration of all three drugs is delayed in renal failure. (From Refs. 78–81, used with permission.)

in renal failure is reduced by one-half to two-thirds of normal, and the elimination half-life is increased by two- and fourfold. These changes are greater than those seen with nondepolarizing muscle relaxants (Table 2).

Although the exact relationship between plasma concentration and effect has not been determined for acetylcholinesterase inhibitors, it seems doubtful that recurarization in patients with renal failure is due to a fall in plasma concentration of the inhibitors without a concurrent fall in plasma concentration of the muscle relaxants.

Of particular interest is the fact that newly transplanted kidneys appear to be as effective as normal kidneys in excreting acetylcholinesterase inhibitors (Table 4) (78–81).

H. Other Factors

Neuromuscular blockade in patients with renal failure may be potentiated and reversal become difficult in the presence of hypokalemia (82), antibiotics such as gentamicin (83) and neomycin, hypermagnesemia (84), hypocalcemia, and antiarrhythmic drugs (85) such as quinidine (86), and furosemide (87).

I. Clinical Management of Patients in Renal Failure

The nondepolarizing muscle relaxant of choice for patients with renal failure would be one with minimal dependence on renal elimination. Atracurium and vecuronium are most appropriate. d-Tubocurarine in small doses is also well tolerated.

The clinician can take the following steps to avoid prolonged paralysis in the patient with renal failure:

1. Apply a peripheral nerve stimulator as a guide to the administration of muscle relaxants.
2. Use potent volatile anesthetic agents (especially isoflurane or enflurane) (88,89) to augment the paralyzing effect of small doses of muscle relaxants.
3. Maintain normal serum electrolyte levels, acid-base status, and body temperature.
4. Avoid drug interaction between muscle relaxants and other drugs such as antibiotics, diuretics, and antiarrhythmics.

Table 4 Pharmacokinetics of Acetylcholinesterase Inhibitors in Normals and Patients with Renal Failure

Drug	Ref.	Patient group	N	Vdss (L/kg)	Cl (ml/kg min)	$t_{1/2}\beta$ (hr)
Neostigmine	79	Normal	8	0.7 ± 0.3	9.0 ± 2.2	1.3 ± 0.8
		Anephric	4	0.8 ± 0.1	3.4 ± 1.3[a]	3.0 ± 0.9[a]
		New transplant	6	1.0 ± 0.5	9.4 ± 2.7	1.7 ± 1.0
Edrophonium	80,81	Normal	4	0.9 ± 0.2	8.2 ± 3.0	1.9 ± 0.8
		Anephric	6	0.8 ± 0.1	2.7 ± 1.4[a]	3.4 ± 1.0[a]
		New transplant	6	0.9 ± 0.2	9.9 ± 2.1	1.4 ± 0.4
Pyridostigmine	80	Normal	5	1.1 ± 0.3	8.6 ± 1.7	1.9 ± 0.2
		Anephric	4	1.0 ± 0.1	2.1 ± 0.6[a]	6.3 ± 2.7[a]
		New transplant	5	1.0 ± 0.2	10.8 ± 2.8	1.4 ± 0.2

All values mean ± SEM.
[a]Significant difference from normal group, $p < 0.05$.

In renal failure, sustained antagonism of nondepolarizing muscle relaxants can be achieved provided some recovery of neuromuscular junction function is present prior to the administration of acetylcholinesterase inhibitors. Close observation is needed in the recovery room in order to detect as early as possible the insidious onset of neuromuscular junction failure caused by drug interaction (e.g., peritoneal absorption of neomycin irrigation fluid).

This author believes that succinylcholine in small doses can also be used safely in patients with renal failure provided hyperkalemia is ruled out prior to its administration.

IV. HEPATIC FAILURE

The pharmacokinetics of nondepolarizing muscle relaxants have been studied in cirrhosis, viral hepatitis, and cholestasis. Resistance and prolonged effect with certain nondepolarizing muscle relaxants have been reported in patients with liver disease.

Cirrhosis is associated with a decrease in number and function of hepatocytes. Hypoproteinemia and renal impairment may also occur. Viral hepatitis compromises the function of hepatocytes, but liver blood flow and biliary excretion remain unimpaired. Cholestasis is characterized by impairment of bile excretion without hepatocytic compromise (although in severe cases, this may not be true).

In this section, the nondepolarizing muscle relaxants will be discussed in order of increasing dependence on liver metabolism and excretion. Unfortunately, studies on the pharmacokinetics of d-tubocurarine, metocurine, and of acetylcholinesterase inhibitors in patients with liver disease are unavailable.

A. Gallamine

The pharmacokinetics of gallamine have been studied in patients with extrahepatic cholestasis (57,90). The clearance and elimination half-life were normal (Table 5). The volume of distribution in one study (90) was normal, but in another (57) it was slightly increased. The onset and duration of action as well as the rate of recovery were normal (57).

Table 5 Pharmacokinetics of Nondepolarizing Muscle Relaxants in Hepatic Failure in Order of Increasing Dependence on the Liver for Elimination

Drug	Ref.	Patient group	N	Vd (L/kg)	Cl (ml/kg min)	$t_{1/2}\beta$ (hr)	Values
Gallamine	90	Normal	4	0.2 ± .04	1.2 ± 0.2	2.7 ± 0.3	Mean ± SEM
		Cholestasis	11	0.2 ± .04	0.9 ± 0.1	3.7 ± 0.7	
Gallamine	56	Normal	17	0.206 ± 0.047	1.2 ± 0.3	2.2 ± 0.6	Mean ± SEM
		Cholestasis	7	0.247 ± 0.022[a]	1.2 ± 0.3	2.6 ± 0.7	
Atracurium[b]	57	Normal	6	0.205 ± 0.054	6.5 ± 1.5	0.37 ± 0.06	Mean ± SD
		Hepatitis	6	0.159 ± 0.021	5.2 ± 0.8	0.35 ± 0.04	
Pancuronium	58	Normal	7	0.26 ± 0.05	1.9 ± 0.6	2.2 ± 0.4	Mean ± SD
		Cholestasis	9	0.31 ± 0.13	1.0 ± 0.3[a]	4.5 ± 1.7[a]	
Pancuronium	90	Normal	12	0.28 ± 0.02	1.8 ± 0.2	2.4 ± 0.3	Mean ± SEM
		Cholestasis	7	0.43 ± 0.06[a]	1.5 ± 0.1	3.7 ± 0.3[a]	
Pancuronium	98	Normal	12	0.28 ± 0.02	1.9 ± 0.1	1.9 ± 0.2	Mean ± SEM
		Cirrhosis	14	0.42 ± 0.06[a]	1.5 ± 0.1[a]	3.4 ± 0.4[a]	
Pancuronium	96	Normal	5	0.20 ± 0.02	1.4 ± 0.3	1.6 ± 0.6	Mean ± SD
		Hepatitis	5	0.21 ± 0.02	0.6 ± 0.2[a]	5.1 ± 3.2[a]	
Vecuronium	98	Normal	9	0.27 ± 0.04	5.0 ± 0.6	0.9 ± 0.1	Mean ± SEM
		Cirrhosis	9	0.23 ± 0.04	2.7 ± 0.5[a]	1,2 ± 0.1[a]	

[a]Significant difference from normal group, $p < 0.05$.
[b]Vd values are calculated Vd_{area}; all others Vdss.

Since gallamine is almost entirely excreted by the kidney, it is not surprising that it has normal pharmacokinetics in patients with cholestasis. Gallamine is an excellent choice for patients with liver disease, provided renal function is preserved.

B. Atracurium

Ward and Neil (58) studied the pharmacokinetics of atracurium in patients with acute liver failure that had been caused by acetaminophen overdose. The patients had also renal failure. Although the volume of distribution of atracurium was increased, its clearance and elimination half-life were normal (Table 5). The unique metabolic pathway of atracurium makes it an ideal drug for patients with hepatic failure. However, as in renal failure (see above), the implications of high blood level of laudanosine in these patients are not known. Indeed, the clinical significance of laudanosine in general is still undetermined.

C. d-Tubocurarine

Resistance to d-tubocurarine has been reported in patients with liver disease (91,92). This phenomenon has been attributed to increased binding of d-tubocurarine to gamma globulin (93,94). In support of this hypothesis are the findings that the ratio of albumin to gamma globulin in liver disease is frequently inverted, and that there is positive correlation between the gamma globulin level in the blood and dose requirement of d-tubocurarine (16,93, 94). However, d-tubocurarine binds plasma proteins only to a limited extent, and therefore, changes in plasma protein levels have minimal effect on its potency (5,12). Moreover, two studies have shown that protein binding of drugs in cirrhotic patients is normal (5,12).

The most likely explanation for the resistance to d-tubocurarine in patients with liver disease is an increase in this drug's volume of distribution. Unfortunately, there are no studies on the pharmacokinetics of d-tubocurarine in these patients.

D. Pancuronium

Pancuronium has been studied extensively in patients with hepatic dysfunction (59,90,95,96) (Table 5). The studies demonstrate that different types of liver disease can affect the disposition of muscle relaxants differently. Two studies showed prolonged elimination half-life and delayed recovery from pancuronium in patients with cholestasis (59,90). In one study (59), a bolus of 6 mg of pancuronium caused paralysis that lasted 114 min in patients with cholestasis versus 70 min in normal subjects. The cause for the long duration of action was different in each of the two studies: Somogyi et al. (59) found a 50% reduction in plasma clearance of pancuronium; Westra et al. (90) found an increase in its volume of distribution. Regardless of the exact mechanism, the evidence is clear that in patients with biliary obstruction, the paralyzing effect of pancuronium is prolonged.

Duvaldestin et al. (95) studied the pharmacokinetics of pancuronium in patients with cirrhosis and found a prolonged distribution half-life, an almost twofold increase in elimination half-life, and a 20% decrease in clearance. This is primarily due to an increase in extracellular fluid, and therefore, in volume of distribution (Table 5). Based on these observations, one would predict that in cirrhotic patients, resistance and increased sensitivity to pancuronium exist at the same time. On one hand, the onset time of pancuronium would be prolonged owing to an increase in the volume of distribution, suggesting resistance to the drug; on the other hand, recovery would be delayed owing to prolonged elimination half-life, suggesting increased sensitivity.

Ward et al. (96) studied the pharmacokinetics of pancuronium in patients with acute hepatic failure and normal renal function. The volume of distribution was normal, but the clearance was reduced by more than one-half, resulting in a threefold increase in elimination half-life. The authors noted that the dose required to produce paralysis was much larger than normal in these patients, implying that the neuromuscular junction was resistant to the effects of pancuronium. This is the only study that suggests altered sensitivity to nondepolarizing muscle relaxants in patients with hepatic disease.

E. Vecuronium

Vecuronium is highly dependent on the liver for metabolism and excretion. It is not surprising, therefore, that the pharmacokinetics of this muscle relaxant are significantly altered in the presence of hepatic failure. In cats, exclusion of blood flow from the liver nearly doubled the duration of action of vecuronium and enhanced its neuromuscular blockade (97).

Duvaldestin (98) studied the pharmacokinetics and pharmacodynamics of vecuronium in patients with cirrhosis and compared them to normal subjects. The volume of distribution of vecuronium in cirrhosis was normal, but the clearance was reduced by roughly 50%. The time interval between the administration of vecuronium and 50% recovery of twitch height was 130 min in patients with cirrhosis versus 62 min in normal subjects. The time to recovery from 25 to 75% of control twitch height was 68 min in cirrhotic patients versus 21 min in normal subjects. Plasma concentration of pancuronium at 50% twitch recovery (Cp_{50}) was similar in both groups (mean values 0.21 and 0.30 μg/ml in normal subjects and cirrhotic patients, respectively, $p > 0.05$). This suggests normal sensitivity to vecuronium in cirrhotic patients.

Duvaldestin (98) remarks that despite the prolonged duration of action of vecuronium in cirrhotic patients, it was still shorter than that of pancuronium in patients free of liver disease.

F. Clinical Management of Patients with Hepatic Failure

Many of the considerations mentioned in Section III.I regarding the clinical management of patients with renal failure apply also to patients with hepatic failure. However, in hepatic failure, the most appropriate nondepolarizing muscle relaxants are gallamine (if renal failure is ruled out) and atracurium because their excretion and degradation are independent of liver function. They do not cause prolonged paralysis in these patients.

As in patients with renal failure, muscle relaxants in patients with liver disease should be given in small doses and titrated to a specific endpoint by using a peripheral nerve stimulator. Onset and duration of paralysis following pancuronium administration may be prolonged owing to increase in volume of distribution. The clinician may have to give a larger initial dose and then wait longer than usual in between "top-up" doses.

The use of potent volatile anesthetics to augment the neuromuscular blockade of small doses of muscle relaxants is recommended. Avoiding drug interactions with antibiotics, antiarrhythmics, and diuretics as well as maintaining normal acid-base status and body temperature can help prevent undesired prolongation of neuromuscular blockade.

REFERENCES

1. Sheiner LB, Stanski DR, Vozeh S, Miller RD, Ham J: Simultaneous modeling of pharmacokinetics and pharmacodynamics: Application to d-tubocurarine. *Clin Pharmacol Ther 25*:358-371, 1979.
2. Matteo RS, Spector S, Horowitz PE: Relation of serum d-tubocurarine concentration to neuromuscular blockade in man. *Anesthesiology 41*:440–443, 1974.
3. Agoston S, Crul JF, Kersten UW, Scaf AHJ: Relationship of the serum concentration of pancuronium to its neuromuscular activity in man. *Anesthesiology 47*:509–512, 1977.
4. Shanks CA, Somogyi AA, Triggs EJ: Dose response and plasma concentration response relationships of pancuronium in man. *Anesthesiology 51*:111–118, 1979.
5. Duvaldestin P, Henzel D: Binding of tubocurarine, fazadinium, pancuronium and Org NC 45 to serum proteins in normal man and in patients with cirrhosis. *Br J Anaesth 54*: 513–516, 1982.
6. Greenblatt DJ, Koch-Weser J: Clinical pharmacokinetics. *N Engl J Med 293*:702–705, 964–970, 1975.
7. Hug CC, Jr: Pharmacokinetics of drugs administered intravenously. *Anesth Analg 57*:704–723, 1978.
8. Hull CJ: Pharmacokinetics and pharmacodynamics. *Br J Anaesth 51*:579–594, 1979.
9. Gibaldi M, Perrier D: *Pharmacokinetics*. Marcel Dekker, New York, 1975.
10. Rowland M, Tozer TN: *Clinical Pharmacokinetics—Concepts and Applications*. Lea & Febiger, Philadelphia, 1980.

11. Stanski DR, Watkins WD: *Drug Disposition in Anesthesia.* Grune & Stratton, New York, 1982.
12. Ghoneim MM, Kramer, Sr E, Bannow R, Pandya H, Routh JI: Binding of d-tubocurarine to plasma proteins in normal man and in patients with hepatic or renal disease. *Anesthesiology 39*:410–415, 1973.
13. Wood M, Stone WJ, Wood AJJ: Plasma binding of pancuronium: Effects of age, sex and disease. *Anesth Analg 62*: 29–32, 1983.
14. Wood M, Wood AJJ: Changes in plasma drug binding and o 1-acid glycoprotein in mother and newborn infant. *Clin Pharmacol. Ther 29*:522–526, 1981.
15. Ghoneim MM, Pandya H: Binding of tubocurarine to specific serum protein fractions. *Br J Anaesth 47*:853–856, 1975.
16. Thompson JM: Pancuronium binding by serum proteins. *Anaesthesia 31*:219–227, 1976.
17. Foldes FF, Deery A: Protein binding of atracurium and other short-acting neuromuscular blocking agents and their interaction with human cholinesterases. *Br J Anaesth 55*:31S–34S, 1983.
18. Bush MT, Alvin JD: Characterization of drug-protein interactions by classic methods. *Ann NY Acad Sci 226*:36, 1973.
19. Cohen, EN, Corbascio A, Fleischli G: The distribution and fate of d-tubocurarine. *J Pharmacol Exp Ther 147*:120–129, 1965.
20. Meijer DKF, Weitering JG, Vermeer GA, Scaf AHJ: Comparative pharmacokinetics of d-tubocurarine and metocurine in man. *Anesthesiology 51*:402–407, 1979.
21. Dal Santo G: Kinetics of distribution of radioactive-labeled muscle relaxants. *Anesthesiology 25*:788–800, 1964.
22. Skivington MA: Protein binding of three tritiated muscle relaxants. *Br J Anaesth 44*:1030–1034, 1972.
23. Olsen GD, Chan EM, Riker WK: Binding of d-tubocurarine di(methyl-^{14}C) ether iodide and other amines to cartilage, chondroitin sulfate and human plasma proteins. *J Pharmacol Exp Ther 195*:242–250, 1975.
24. Chagas C: *The Fate of Curare During Curarization: Ciba Foundation Symposium on Curare and Curarelike Agents* (Reucks AVS, ed.), Little, Brown, Boston, pp. 2–32, 1972.

25. Waser P: Localization of ^{14}C-pancuronium by histo- and whole body-autoradiography in normal and pregnant mice. *Naunyn Schmeidebergs Arch Pharmacol 279*:399–412, 1973.
26. Gibaldi M, Levy G, Hayton W: Kinetics of the elimination and neuromuscular blocking effect of d-tubocurarine in man. *Anesthesiology 36*:213–218, 1972.
27. Brotherton WP, Matteo RS: Pharmacokinetics and pharmacodynamics of metocurine in humans with and without renal failure. *Anesthesiology 55*:273–276, 1981.
28. Matteo RS, Nishateno K, Pua EK, Spector S: Pharmacokinetics of d-tubocurarine in man: Effect of an osmotic diuretic on urinary excretion. *Anesthesiology 52*:335–338, 1980.
29. Agoston S, Crul JF, Kersten UW, Houwertjes MC, Scaaf AHJ: The relationship between disposition and duration of action of a congeneric of steroidal neuromuscular blocking agents. *Acta Anaesth Scand 21*:24–30, 1977.
30. Bencini A, Scaf AHJ, Sohn YJ, Kersten U, Agoston S: Clinical pharmacokinetics of vecuronium, in *Clinical Experiences with Norcuron (Org NC 45 Vecuronium Bromide)* (Agoston S, Bowman WC, Miller RD, Viby-Mogensen J, eds.), Excerpta Medica, Amsterdam, pp. 115–123, 1983.
31. Stenlake JB, Waigh RD, Urwin J, Dewar GH, Cohen GG: Atracurium conception and inception. *Br J Anaesth 55*: 3S–10S, 1983.
32. Neill EAM, Chapple DJ: Metabolic studies in the cat with atracurium: A neuromuscular blocking agent designed for non-enzymatic inactivation at physiological pH. *Xenobiotica 12*:203, 1982.
33. Agoston S, Vermeer GA, Kersten UW, Meijer DKF: The fate of pancuronium bromide in man. *Acta Anaesth Scan 17*: 267–275, 1973.
34. Miller RD, Agoston S, Booij LHDJ, Kersten UW, Crul JF, Ham J: The comparative potency and pharmacokinetics of pancuronium and its metabolites in anesthetized man. *J Pharmacol Exp Ther 207*:539–543, 1978.
35. Savage DS, Sleigh T, Carlyle I: The emergence of Org NC 45 from the pancuronium series. *Br J Anaesth 52*:3S–9S, 1980.

36. Somogyi AA, Shanks CA, Triggs EJ: The effect of renal failure on the disposition and neuromuscular blocking action of pancuronium bromide. *Europ J Clin Pharmacol 12*: 23-29, 1977.
37. Marshall IG, Gibb AJ, Durant NN: Neuromuscular and vagal blocking actions of pancuronium bromide, its metabolites, and vecuronium bromide (Org NC 45) and its potential metabolites in the anesthetized cat. *Br J Anaesth 55*:703-714, 1983.
38. Agoston S, Vermeer GA, Kersten UW, Scaf AHJ: A preliminary investigation of the renal and hepatic excretion of gallamine triethiodide in man. *Br J Anaesth 50*:345-350, 1978.
39. Roberts JB, Thomas BH, Wilson A: Distribution and excretion of ^{14}C-neostigmine in the rat and hen. *Br J Pharmacol Chemother 25*:234-242, 1965.
40. Meijer DKF, Weitering JG, Vonk, RJ: Hepatic uptake and biliary excretion of d-tubocurarine and trimethyltubocurarine in the rat in vivo and in isolated perfused rat livers. *J Pharmacol Exp Ther 198*:229-239, 1976.
41. Vonk RJ, Scholtens E, Keulemans GTP, Meijer DKF: Choleresis and transport mechanisms: i.v. influence of bile salt choleresis on the hepatic transport of the organic cations d-tubocurarine and 4N-acetylprocaine ethobromide. *Naunyn Schmiedebergs Arch Pharmacol 302*:1-7, 1978.
42. Weitering JG, Lammers W, Meijer DKF, Mulder GJ: Localization of d-tubocurarine in rat liver lysosomes: Lysosomal uptake, biliary excretion and displacement by quinacrine in vivo. *Naunyn Schmiedebergs Arch Pharmacol 299*:277-281, 1977.
43. Meijer DKF, Scaf AHJ: Inhibition of the transport of d-tubocurarine from blood to bile by k-strophantoside in the isolated perfused rat liver. *Eur J Pharmacol 4*:343-346, 1968.
44. Westra P, Houwertes MC, Wesseling H, Meijer DKF: Bile salts and neuromuscular blocking agents. *Br J Anaesth 53*:407-415, 1981.
45. Feldman SA, Cohen EN, and Golling RC: The excretion of gallamine in the dog. *Anesthesiology 30*:593-598, 1969.

46. Duvaldestin P, Saada J, Berger JL, D'Hollander A, Desmonts JM: Pharmacokinetics, pharmacodynamics, and dose-response relationships of pancuronium in control and elderly subjects. *Anesthesiology 56*:36–40, 1982.
47. Upton RA, Nguyen T-L, Miller RD, Castagnoli N Jr: Renal and biliary elimination of vecuronium (Org NC 45) and pancuronium in rats. *Anesth Analg 61*:313–316, 1982.
48. Fahey MR, Morris RB, Miller RD, Nguyen T-L, Upton RA: Pharmacokinetics of Org NC 45 (Norcuron®) in patients with and without renal failure. *Br J Anaesth 53*:1049–1053, 1981.
49. Weatherley BC, Williams SG, Neill EAM: Pharmacokinetics, pharmacodynamics and dose-response relationships of atracurium administered i.v. *Br J Anaesth 55*:395–455, 1983.
50. Fahey MR, Rupp SM, Fisher DM, Miller RD, Sharma M, Canfell C, Castagnoli K, Hennis PJ: The pharmacokinetics and pharmacodynamics of atracurium in patients with and without renal failure. *Anesthesiology 61*:699–702, 1984.
51. Van der Veen F, Bencini A: Pharmacokinetics and pharmacodynamics of Org NC 45 in man. *Br J Anaesth 52*:37S–41S, 1980.
52. Riordan DD, Gilbertson AA: Prolonged curarization in a patient with renal failure. Case report. *Br J Anaesth 43*: 506–507, 1971.
53. Churchill-Davidson HC, Way WL, deJong RH: The muscle relaxants and renal excretion. *Anesthesiology 28*:540–546, 1967.
54. Rouse JM, Galley RLA, Bevan DR: Prolonged curarization following renal transplantation: A retrospective study. *Anaesthesia 32*:247–251, 1977.
55. Miller RD, Cullen DJ: Renal failure and postoperative respiratory failure: recurarization? *Br J Anaesth 48*:253–256, 1976.
56. McLeod K, Watson MJ, Rawlins MD: Pharmacokinetics of pancuronium in patients with normal and impaired renal function. *Br J Anaesth 48*:341–345, 1976.
57. Ramzan MI, Shanks CA, Triggs EJ: Pharmacokinetics and pharmacodynamics of gallamine triethiodide in patients with total biliary obstruction. *Anesth Analg 60*:289–296, 1981.

58. Ward S, Neill EAM: Pharmacokinetics of atracurium in acute hepatic failure (with acute renal failure). *Br J Anaesth 55*: 1169–1172, 1983.
59. Somogyi AA, Shanks CA, Triggs EJ: Disposition kinetics of pancuronium bromide in patients with total biliary obstruction. *Br J Anaesth 49*:1103–1107, 1977.
60. Buzello W, Agoston S: Kinetics of intercompartmental disposition and excretion of tubocurarine, gallamine, alcuronium and pancuronium in patients with normal and impaired renal function. *Anaesthetist 27*:319–321, 1978.
61. Hunter JM, Jones RS, Utting JE: Use of atracurium in patients with no renal function. *Br J Anaesth 54*:1251–1258, 1982.
62. Fahey MR, Rupp SM, Canfell C, Fisher DM, Miller RD, Sharma M, Castagnoli K, Hennis PJ: The effect of renal failure on laudanosine excretion in man. *Br J Anaesth 57*: 1049–1051, 1985.
63. Mercier J, Mercier E: Action de quelques alcaloides secondaires de l'opium sur l'electrocorticogramme du chien. *C R Soc Biol (Paris) 149*:760–762, 1955.
64. Babel A: Etude comparative de la laudanosine et de la papaveine au point de vue pharmacodynamique. *Rev Med Suisse Romande 19*:657–688, 1899.
65. Shi WZ, Fahey MR, Fisher DM, Miller RD, Canfell C, Eger EI: Laudanozine (a metabolite of atracurium) increases the minimum alveolar concentration of halothane in rabbits. *Anesthesiology 63*:584–588, 1985.
66. Lanier WL, Milde JH, Michenfelder JD: The cerebral effects of pancuronium and atracurium in halothane-anesthetized dogs. *Anesthesiology 63*:589–597, 1985.
67. Cohen EN, Brewer HW, Smith D: The metabolism and elimination of d-tubocurarine-HX*3X. *Anesthesiology 28*:309–317, 1967.
68. Miller RD, Stevens WC, Way WL: The effect of renal failure and hyperkalemia on the duration of pancuronium neuromuscular blockade in man. *Anesth Analg 52*:661–666, 1973.
69. Lavine LM, Hindein BI: Hemodialysis as treatment for prolonged neuromuscular blockade in anephric patients. *Anesthesiology 59*:264, 1983.

70. Abrams RE, Hornbein TF: Inability to reverse pancuronium blockade in a patient with renal failure and hepatic disease. *Anesthesiology 42*:362–364, 1975.
71. Fairley HB: Prolonged intercostal paralysis due to a relaxant. *Br Med J 2*:986, 1950.
72. Joske RA, Ebeling P, Stanistreet RH: Delayed post-operative recurarization. *Med J Aust 1*:856–859, 1954.
73. Montgomery JB, Bennett-Jones N: Gallamine triethiodide and renal disease. *Lancet 2*:1243–1244, 1956.
74. Jenkins IR: Three cases of apparent recurarization. *Br J Anaesth 33*:314–318, 1961.
75. Feldman SA: Effect of changes in electrolytes, hydration and pH upon the reactions to muscle relaxants. *Br J Anaesth 35*: 546–551, 1963.
76. White RD, DeWeerd JH, Dawson B: Gallamine in anesthesia for patients with chronic renal failure undergoing bilateral nephrectomy. *Anesth Analg 50*:11–16, 1971.
77. Gibaldi M, Levy G, Hayton WL: Tubocurarine and renal function. *Br J Anaesth 44*:163–165, 1972.
78. Cronnelly R, Stanski DR, Miller RD, Sheiner, RD: Pyridostigmine kinetics with and without renal function. *Clin Pharmacol Ther 28*:78–81, 1980.
79. Cronnelly R, Stanski DR, Miller RD, Sheiner LB, Sohn YJ: Renal function and the pharmacokinetics of neostigmine in anesthetized man. *Anesthesiology 51*:222–226, 1979.
80. Morris RB, Cronnelly R, Miller RD, Stanski DR, Fahey MR: Pharmacokinetics of edrophonium in anephric and renal transplant patients. *Br J Anaesth 53*:1311–1314, 1981.
81. Morris RB, Cronnelly R, Miller RD, Stanski DR, Fahey MR: Pharmacokinetics of edrophonium and neostigmine when antagonizing d-tubocurarine neuromuscular blockade in man. *Anesthesiology 54*:399–402, 1981.
82. Feldman SA, Levi JA: Prolonged paresis following gallamine: A case report. *Br J Anaesth 35*:804–806, 1963.
83. Regan AG, Perumbetti PPV: Pancuronium and gentamicin interaction in patients with renal failure (letter). *Anesth Analg 59*:393, 1980.
84. Ghoneim MM, Long JP: The interaction between magnesium and other neuromuscular blocking agents. *Anesthesiology 32*: 23–27, 1970.

85. Harrah MD, Way WL, Katzung BG: The interaction of d-tubocurarine with antiarrhythmic drugs. *Anesthesiology 33*:406–410, 1970.
86. Miller RD, Way WI, Katzung BG: The potentiation of neuromuscular blocking agents by quinidine. *Anesthesiology 28*: 1036–1041, 1967.
87. Miller RD, Sohn YS, Matteo RS: Enhancement of d-tubocurarine neuromuscular blockade by diuretics in man. *Anesthesiology 45*:442–445, 1976.
88. Rupp SM, Miller RD, Gencarelli PJ: Vecuronium-induced neuromuscular blockade during enflurane, isoflurane, and halothane anesthesia in humans. *Anesthesiology 60*:102–105, 1984.
89. Rupp SM, McChristian JW, Miller RD: Neuromuscular effects of atracurium during halothane-nitrous oxide and enflurane-nitrous oxide anesthesia in humans. *Anesthesiology 63*: 16–19, 1985.
90. Westra P, Vermeer GA, deLange AR, Scaf AHJ, Meijer DKF, Wesseling H: Hepatic and renal disposition of pancuronium and gallamine in patients with extrahepatic cholestasis. *Br J Anaesth 53*:331–338, 1981.
91. Dundee JW, Gray TC: Resistance to d-tubocurarine chloride in the presence of liver damage. *Lancet 2*:16–17, 1953.
92. El-Hakim MS, Baraka A: d-Tubocurarine in liver disease. *Kasr el Aini J Surg 4*:99, 1963.
93. Baraka A, Gabali F: Correlation between tubocurarine requirements and plasma protein pattern. *Br J Anaesth 40*: 89–93, 1968.
94. Stovner J, Theodorsen L, Bjelke E: Sensitivity to tubocurarine and alcuronium with special reference to plasma protein pattern. *Br J Anaesth 43*:385–391, 1971.
95. Duvaldestin P, Agoston S, Henzel D, Kersten UW, Desmonts JM: Pancuronium pharmacokinetics in patients with liver cirrhosis. *Br J Anaesth 50*:1131–1136, 1978.
96. Ward S, Judge S, Corall I: Pharmacokinetics pancuronium bromide in liver failure. *Br J Anaesth 54*:227P, 1982.
97. Durant NN, Houwertjes MC, Agoston S: Hepatic elimination of Org NC45 and pancuronium. *Anesthesiology 51*:S267, 1979.

98. Duvaldestin P, Berger JL, Videcoq M, Desmonts JM: Pharmacokinetics and pharmacodynamics of Org NC45 in patients with cirrhosis. *Anesthesiology 57*:A238, 1982.
99. Ramzan MI, Shanks CA, Triggs EJ: Pharmacokinetic of tubocurarine administered by combined i.v. bolus and infusion. *Br J Anaesth 52*:893–899, 1980.
100. Somogyi AA, Shanks CA, Triggs EJ: Clinical pharmacokinetics of pancuronium bromide. *Eur J Clin Pharmacol 10*:367-372, 1976.
101. Ramzan MI, Triggs EJ, Shanks CA: Pharmacokinetic studies in man with gallamine triethiodide. I. Single and multiple clinical doses. *Eur J Clin Pharmacol 17*:135–143, 1980.

7
Nondepolarizing Muscle Relaxants in Burned Patients

NISHAN G. GOUDSOUZIAN
Harvard Medical School, and Massachusetts General Hospital, Boston, Massachusetts

J. A. JEEVENDRA MARTYN
Shriners Burn Institute, and Massachusetts General Hospital, Boston, Massachusetts

I. INTRODUCTION

Burned patients present a unique challenge to the anesthesiologist. Thermal injuries stress the cardiovascular and pulmonary systems (1-3) and alter hepatic and renal function. The latter may affect the metabolism of drugs (4-6). The situation is further compounded by the continuous state of catabolism and multiple exposures to drugs and anesthetic agents, which are commonly used in the management of burned patients. Often, all this ends in multiorgan dysfunction (6,7).

Muscle relaxants are important to the anesthetic management of burned patients during both the acute and chronic phases of recovery. Muscle relaxants are used for tracheal intubation, for surgical relaxation, and to facilitate mechanical ventilation in critically burned patients. Because of hepatic and renal complications, the pharmacokinetics and pharmacodynamics of muscle relaxants are altered.

The response of burned patients to succinylcholine is reviewed elsewhere in this book (see Chap. IV). This chapter reviews the pharmacology of nondepolarizing muscle relaxants in burned patients, and provides guidelines for their clinical use.

II. PHARMACOLOGY

A. Dose Requirements

Studies in recent years have established that burned patients are very resistant to nondepolarizing muscle relaxants (8-11). In severely burned children (Table 1), we have found that $ED_{50\%}$ and $ED_{95\%}$ of pancuronium (the dose that causes 50 and 95% twitch depression, respectively) is 0.08 and 0.13 mg/kg,

Table 1 The $ED_{50\%}$, $ED_{95\%}$ (mg/kg), and Recovery Time (min) (5–25% of Control) of d-Tubocurarine, Metocurine, and Pancuronium in Burned (B) and Unburned (U) Patients

Ref.	Relaxant	Anesthesia	% Burn	$ED_{50\%}$		$ED_{95\%}$		Recovery time	
				B	U	B	U	B	U
9[a]	d-Tubocurarine	N_2O-Narcotic	25–50	0.78	0.26	1.8	0.51	—	—
10[b]	Metocurine	N_2O-Narcotic	35	0.2–1.2	0.15	0.6–4	0.32	29	28
11[b]	Metocurine	N_2O-Narcotic	42 ± 39	0.23	0.15	0.81	0.32	30	29
8[b]	Pancuronium	N_2O-Narcotic	—	0.08	0.03	0.13	0.05	26	16

[a]Study in adults.
[b]Study in children.

respectively. This is well above the doses for unburned patients of 0.031 and 0.054 mg/kg, respectively (8). A pronounced resistance has also been observed in burned adult patients: The $ED_{50\%}$ and $ED_{95\%}$ of d-tubocurarine were 0.7 and 1.8 mg/kg, respectively, whereas in unburned patients the values were 0.26 and 0.51 mg/kg, respectively. Similar resistance has been observed with the nondepolarizing muscle relaxant metocurine (10,11). When compared to unburned patients, the dose-response curves for nondepolarizing muscle relaxants in burned patients are shifted to the right (Fig. 1), thus indicating their resistance.

The degree of resistance to nondepolarizing muscle relaxants depends upon the extent of the burn (Fig. 2) and the duration of time since it occurred (10,11). When the burn covers $<10\%$ of body surface area, the patient shows no resistance to muscle relaxants. When it covers $>40\%$ of body surface area, the dose requirements increase by two and one-half- to threefold. Patients with intermediate-size burns show a moderate increase in dose requirement.

The resistance to nondepolarizing muscle relaxants is not seen until a few days after the burn was sustained. The peak resistance is observed about 2 weeks later, and it persists for several weeks. Patients with major burns may remain resistant to muscle relaxants even after the burns have healed completely (10). Although the resistance decreases with time, it may linger for as long as 2 years after the burn was sustained.

B. Pharmacokinetics

An early theory on the possible cause of resistance to muscle relaxants in burned patients was that these agents ooze from the body through the raw surfaces of the skin, as has been shown to occur with some antibiotics (12). However, pharmacodynamic and pharmacokinetic studies with d-tubocurarine refuted this speculation (Fig. 3, p. 198). The elimination half-lives and clearance of d-tubocurarine are rather similar in burned and unburned patients (13) (Table 2).

In burned patients, renal excretion at 24 hr after its administration and central volume of distribution of d-tubocurarine were greater than normal. However, no differences were found

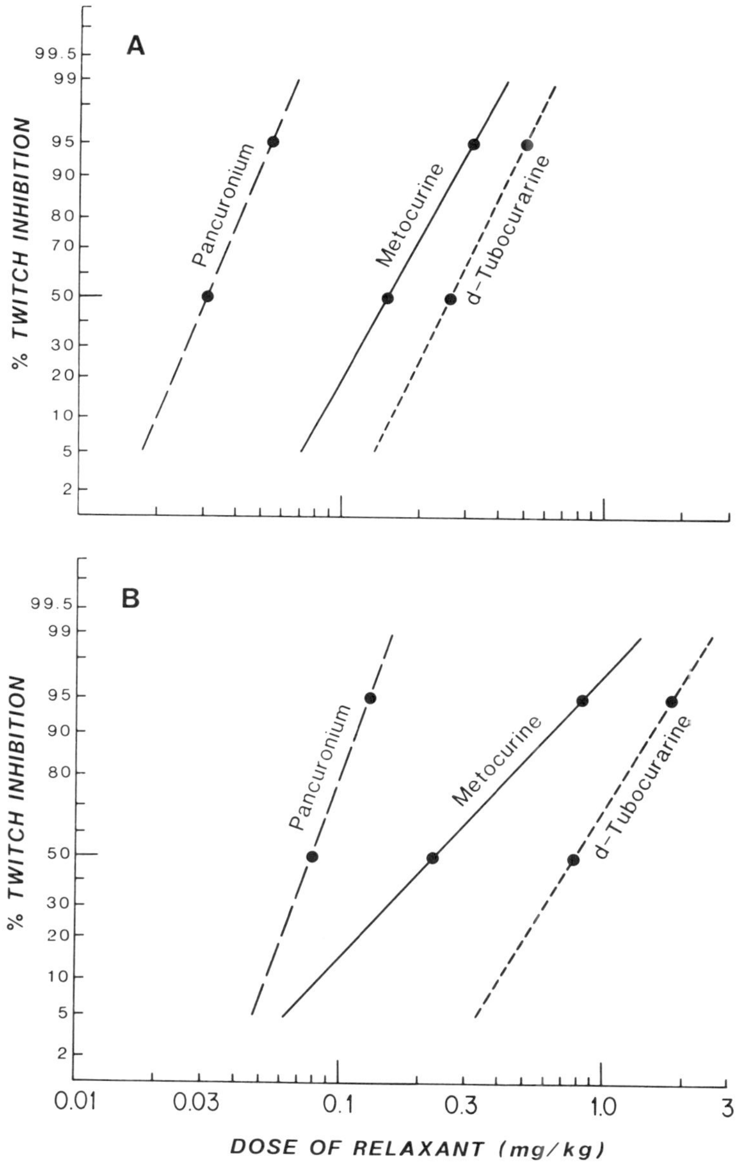

Figure 1 Dose-response curves of d-tubocurarine, metocurine, and pancuronium in control (A) and burned (B) patients. Note the marked shift to the right of all curves in the burned patients. (From Refs. 8, 9, and 11, used with permission.)

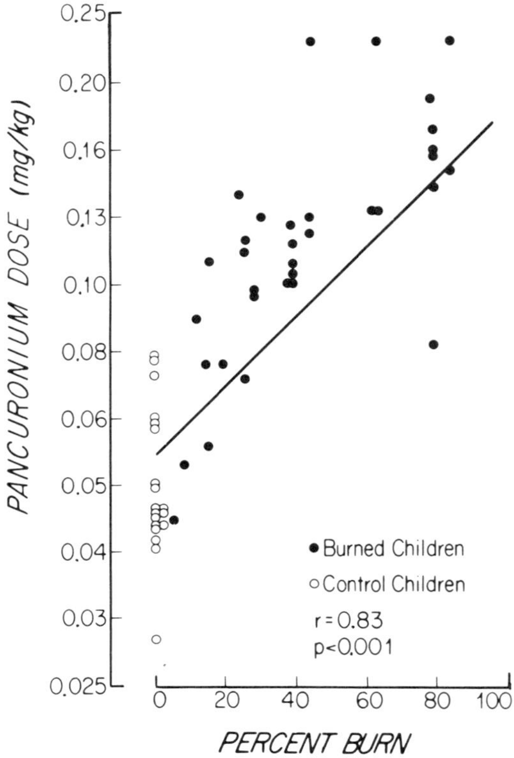

Figure 2 The correlation between log $ED_{95\%}$ and magnitude of burn. Note the good correlation between the two. The regression line is described by the equation: log $ED_{95\%}$ = 0.00641 x % burn - 1.256. (Modified from Ref. 8, used with permission.)

at 6 hr after its administration, and, therefore, the kinetic differences could not account for the resistance to muscle relaxants during surgery in burned patients.

The rate of recovery of burned patients from muscle relaxants varies and depends on the individual muscle relaxant. Following administration of pancuronium, the recovery time of twitch response from 5 to 25% was 24.5 min and 16.1 min ($p < 0.008$) in burned and in unburned pediatric patients,

Table 2 Pharmacokinetic Parameters of d-Tubocurarine in Burned and Unburned Patients. Note the Major Differences in the Unbound Initial Volume of Distribution and the 24-hr Urinary Excretion

Pharmacokinetic parameters	Burned patients	Unburned patients
Distribution half-life (min)	3.9	4.2
Elimination half-life (hr)	6.5	6.2
Initial volume of distribution (L/kg)	0.037	0.028
Total volume of distribution (L/kg)	0.28	0.42
Total clearance (ml/kg min)	0.53	0.77[a]
Calculated % protein bound	67	50
Unbound initial volume of distribution (L/kg)	0.11	0.06[a]
Unbound total volume of distribution (L/kg)	0.86	0.96
Unbound (intrinsic) clearance (ml/kg/min)	1.62	1.56
Urinary excretion in 6 hr, %	37.7	27.7
Urinary excretion in 24 hr, %	57.4	40.2[a]

Source: From Ref. 14, used with permission.

respectively (8). The recovery time from d-tubocurarine and metocurine, however, were normal (9,11).

One may speculate that the difference in recovery time between muscle relaxants in burned patients is due to the differences in the metabolism of these drugs. Normally, metocurine and d-tubocurarine are excreted unchanged, mostly by the kidneys (14), and their elimination is independent of liver function. Pancuronium, on the other hand, undergoes a certain degree of metabolism in the liver. Its elimination, therefore, is more susceptible to liver dysfunction. Since thermal injuries and multiple drug exposures in burned patients have been shown to depress liver drug metabolism (3,5), this may explain the longer recovery time from pancuronium when compared to d-tubocurarine and metocurine.

C. Protein Binding

Protein binding apparently plays a significant role in the resistance of burned patients to nondepolarizing muscle relaxants. d-Tubocurarine undergoes 70% more protein binding in burned patients than in unburned patients. The protein binding peaks at 1–2 weeks after the thermal injury occurred and coincides with the onset of clinical resistance to the muscle relaxants. However, the increase in protein binding can account only partially for the resistance observed (11,15). The increase in protein binding is probably due to a rise in the blood level of alpha$_1$-acid glycoprotein, a globulin component which is released by the liver in burned patients.

III. CHANGES AT THE NEUROMUSCULAR JUNCTION

Animal studies have shown that in certain neuromuscular disorders, particularly following muscle denervation, there is an increase in the number of extrajunctional acetylcholine receptors in the muscle membrane and a change in their binding properties (16). Normally, the acetylcholine receptors are concentrated at the neuromuscular junction itself, and only a few may be found extrajunctionally, incorporated in the muscle membrane.

Following muscle denervation, there is a five- to 30-fold increase in the number of extrajunctional receptors, and eventually the receptors spread over the entire muscle fiber membrane. This becomes apparent about 2 days after denervation, it peaks within 1–3 weeks, and declines gradually over a long period of time (17–19). The density of extrajunctional receptors is significantly lower than that of junctional receptors (100–600 vs. up to 20,000 receptors per square micrometer, respectively) (20). A similar spread of extrajunctional receptors can also be found following prolonged immobilization and in embryonic skeletal muscles.

Extrajunctional receptors have loose attachment to the muscle membrane. Physiologically, they respond like junctional receptors: They interact with acetylcholine and undergo depolarization, and they have specific binding sites for alpha-bungarotoxins. Following depolarization, however, the channels in extrajunctional acetylcholine receptors remain open for a longer period of time (21) and the current generated by these channels is weaker. Three times the normal dose of d-tubocurarine is required to block all the extrajunctional receptors of a denervated muscle (19).

Since patients with denervated or immobilized muscles are resistant to nondepolarizing muscle relaxants (20,22), presumably because of the extrajunctional receptors, it is possible that the resistance to muscle relaxants in burned patients is also due to an extrajunctional spread of acetylcholine receptors in thermally injured muscles. Attempts to assess the extrajunctional spread of receptors in thermally injured muscles have been unsuccessful because experimentally burned animals die before these receptors appear.

An increase in the number of extrajunctional acetylcholine receptors would explain not only the resistance to nondepolarizing muscle relaxants, but also the release of potassium and resultant hyperkalemia following the administration of succinylcholine that is observed in burned patients (23,24).

Another possible reason for the resistance to nondepolarizing muscle relaxants in burned patients could be the significant rise in catecholamine levels in these patients. Standaert has shown that agents which increase cyclic adenosine monophosphate (AMP) activity, such as theophylline, cause an increase in acetylcholine release (25). This in turn increases resistance to nondepolarizing muscle relaxants. Theophylline has also been shown to reverse the neuromuscular-blocking effect of nondepolarizing muscle relaxants in man (26). Since catecholamines increase cyclic AMP activity, the rise in catecholamine levels in burned patients could possibly be the cause for the resistance to muscle relaxants in these patients. There is, however, no direct evidence for this.

IV. MONITORING THE NEUROMUSCULAR JUNCTION

Monitoring the neuromuscular junction in burned patients often presents a problem because the hands and the forearms of the patient may be involved in the thermal injury. Nevertheless, we have usually been successful in monitoring burned patients, particularly when the burn is superficial. We use subcutaneous needles as stimulating electrodes and record the contraction of the abductor pollicis. There has been good correlation between the information obtained from the monitor and the clinical signs of relaxation.

If both arms and hands are badly damaged, the legs can be used instead by stimulating the posterior tibial nerve and recording the contraction of flexor hallucis longus. However, a certain quantitative difference may exist in the results between leg and hand monitoring. Observing the contractions of the orbicularis oculi in response to facial nerve stimulation may also be a useful guide to the administration of muscle relaxants. Quantitative information can be obtained by using train-of-four stimulation and counting the number of visible muscle contractions.

V. REVERSAL OF MUSCLE RELAXANTS

Despite the relatively high doses of muscle relaxants, the neuromuscular blockade in burn patients is easily reversible. The usual doses of neostigmine and atropine provide adequate reversal, as confirmed by neuromuscular junction monitoring. We have observed no evidence of "recurarization" in our patients, regardless of their general clinical condition.

Burned patients are often critically ill and many require postoperative mechanical ventilation. This is particularly true if they are hypothermic, have lost large amounts of blood and other fluids, or have cardiopulmonary complications. In such cases, it is advisable not to reverse the neuromuscular blockade. The tracheal tube should be left in place and mechanical ventilation should be administered in order to reduce the patient's metabolic requirements.

VI. TRACHEAL INTUBATION

A. Intubation Without the Use of Muscle Relaxants

There is no standard approach to the tracheal intubation of burned patients. Succinylcholine is definitely contraindicated (see Chap. IV). Although deep inhalation anesthesia can be used to facilitate intubation, these patients may not tolerate it because of their compromised cardiovascular systems (27–30). In addition, in the presence of facial burns, it may be difficult to assess the depth of anesthesia. This may lead to premature attempts at intubation, complicated by retching, vomiting, and laryngospasm.

Laryngospasm and pulmonary aspiration of gastric contents are particularly dangerous in burned patients because of their increased metabolic needs. Also, because the immune system is often depressed, recovery from aspiration pneumonia is protracted. When possible, awake intubation is preferable, although this may prove difficult to achieve in pediatric patients.

B. Intubation Facilitated by Long-Acting Muscle Relaxants

Since succinylcholine is contraindicated and deep general anesthesia is poorly tolerated in burned patients (27–30), the use of nondepolarizing muscle relaxants for tracheal intubation should be considered. Several agents are available. By tailoring the agent and dose to the needs of the individual patient, tracheal intubation can be achieved safely.

The discovery that combinations of pancuronium and metocurine, or pancuronium and d-tubocurarine, are more potent than equivalent doses of these muscle relaxants given individually (31) was a significant contribution to the practice of anesthesia. This mutual potentiation of muscle relaxants has been shown in unburned (31) as well as in burned patients (32).

The administration of muscle relaxants in combinations has several significant advantages over the administration of individual muscle relaxants alone:

1. The dose requirement of each relaxant in the mixture is reduced by half when compared to the equivalent dose of each individual muscle relaxant given alone (Table 3). A combination of muscle relaxants, therefore, allows quicker recovery from the same level of neuromuscular blockade.
2. The side effects of a combination of muscle relaxants are diminished because of the smaller dose of each individual muscle relaxant in the combination.
3. The onset time (time to maximum effect) of a combination is markedly shorter than that of an equivalent dose of an individual muscle relaxant given alone.

Burned patients often have paralytic gastrointestinal distention, and are in serious danger of pulmonary aspiration of gastric contents during induction of general anesthesia, and therefore securing the airway in these patients is of paramount importance. The most commonly used method to secure the airway in patients who are in danger of pulmonary aspiration is rapid tracheal intubation. Succinylcholine is usually the muscle relaxant of choice because of its rapid onset, but as underscored above, this drug is absolutely contraindicated in burned patients (see also Chap. IV).

In search of alternatives, we studied the effect of one intubating dose-equivalent of pancuronium ($2 \times ED_{95}$ 0.07 mg/kg) combined with one intubating dose-equivalent of metocurine (0.25 mg/kg) (33) and found that the onset time was 3 min. Increasing the doses of muscle relaxants in the combination to three effective dose-equivalents (pancuronium, 0.1 mg/kg, and metocurarine, 0.37 mg/kg) further shortened the onset time to 1.3 min, almost as short as that of succinylcholine.

The duration of action of a combination of three effective dose-equivalents of pancuronium and metocurine was about 2.5 hr (Table 3). Since most surgical procedures in burned patients are

Table 3 Summary of Data on the Use of Combinations of Muscle Relaxants in Burned Patients

Clinical condition	Dose	Combinations[a] (mg/kg) P + M	Recovery time (min) to 25% twitch response
Unburned	$ED_{95\%}$	0.013 + 0.051	15
Acute mild burn	$ED_{95\%}$	0.025 + 0.1	17
Acute severe	$ED_{95\%}$	0.040 + 0.16	23
Reconstructive	2 x $ED_{95\%}$	0.030 + 0.1	46
Acute burn	2 x $ED_{95\%}$	0.070 + 0.25	113
Reconstructive	3 x $ED_{95\%}$	0.045 + 0.1	86
Acute	3 x $ED_{95\%}$	0.100 + 0.37	152

Abbreviations: P, pancuronium; M, metocurine.

[a]It was assumed that relaxant equivalents for pancuronium and metocurine were 5 and 20 μg/kg, respectively.

Source: From Refs. 32 and 33, used with permission.

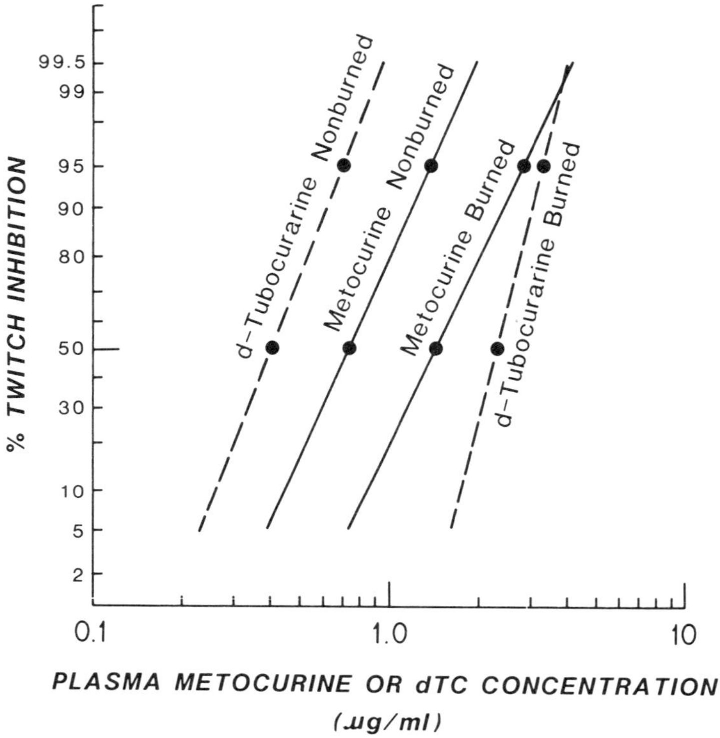

Figure 3 Plasma level of d-tubocurarine and metocurine during recovery plotted against twitch depression in burned and unburned patients. Note the shift to the right of the curves in the burned patients.

prolonged, the duration of action induced by this combination is acceptable. Combining nondepolarizing muscle relaxants, therefore, is a satisfactory alternative to succinylcholine for rapid tracheal intubation. However, the patient's airway should be carefully assessed prior to the administration of the muscle relaxants. If difficult intubation is anticipated, muscle relaxants should be avoided and the airway secured while the patient is breathing spontaneously.

C. Intermediate-Acting Muscle Relaxants

The introduction to clinical practice of the intermediate-acting muscle relaxants, atracurium and vecuronium, offers new means of muscle relaxation for burned patients (33). These muscle relaxants have minimal cardiovascular side effects, although atracurium in large doses releases histamine and may cause transient hypotension (34). It is not clear whether histamine release in burned patients poses a particular problem; as a matter of fact, we have used larger doses of atracurium in these subjects without any untoward effects.

Preliminary experience with atracurium indicates that burned patients are resistant to this muscle relaxant, as they are to the long-acting muscle relaxants. Large doses of atracurium (1–2 mg/kg) or vecuronium (0.25–0.5 mg/kg) are needed in burned patients even for short surgical procedures. Atracurium may be particularly useful for burned patients in renal and liver failures because it is metabolized spontaneously by Hofmann elimination and ester hydrolysis (34), and it is completely independent of hepatic and renal excretions.

Future studies will determine whether the intermediate-acting muscle relaxants are practical and useful drugs in burned patients.

VII. CLINICAL USE OF MUSCLE RELAXANTS

A. Long-Acting Muscle Relaxants

The choice of a muscle relaxant for a particular burned patient should depend primarily on the patient's cardiovascular state and renal and hepatic functions. Particular attention should be paid to the cardiovascular system when the burns cover 40% or more of the patient's body surface area.

In our practice, we most often use a mixture of pancuronium and metocurine, 0.07 and 0.25 mg/kg of each, respectively. For patients with extensive burns who are scheduled for lengthy surgical procedures, we use pancuronium and metocurine in incremental doses, up to 0.1 and 0.375 mg/kg of each, respectively. The onset time of such a combination is 90 sec. This combination may also be given as a bolus for rapid tracheal intubation, although it may cause minor cardiovascular changes.

We tend to avoid pancuronium in tachycardic patients and administer instead 1–1.5 mg/kg of d-tubocurarine, or 1 mg/kg of metocurine (two to three times the normal dose). In patients with impaired renal function, we tend to use d-tubocurarine, and in patients with impaired liver function, metocurine. If the patient's cardiovascular system is unstable, we prefer to use pancuronium because it stimulates the circulation by its vagolytic effect and by releasing catecholamines.

B. Intermediate-Acting Muscle Relaxants

The intermediate-acting muscle relaxants are useful in burned patients with relatively small burns who require short surgical procedures. Higher doses than usual are necessary. Because of the relatively short duration of action of the intermediate-acting muscle relaxants, monitoring the neuromuscular junction for the purpose of titration of the neuromuscular blockade is recommended.

Except when postoperative ventilatory support is indicated, the neuromuscular blockade should be reversed at the conclusion of surgery. Rapid and complete recovery of all muscle power is essential in burned patients because of their enormous metabolic requirements.

REFERENCES

1. Martyn JAJ, Snider MT, Szyfelbein SK, et al.: Right ventricular dysfunction following thermal injury. *Ann Surg 191*: 330–335, 1980.
2. Szyfelbein SK: Modern trends in burn care. *J Roy Soc Med 75*:26–32, 1982.
3. Martyn JAJ, Szyfelbein SK: Pathophysiology and management of burn trauma in children. *Semin Anesth 3*:75–97, 1984.
4. Moncrief JA: Burns. *N Engl J Med 288*:444–454, 1973.

5. Martyn JAJ, Greenblatt DJ, Quinby WC: Diazepam kinetics in patients with severe burns. *Anesth Analg 62*:293–297, 1982.
6. Martyn JAJ, Greenblatt DJ, Abernethy DR: Increased cimetidine clearance in burned patients. *JAMA 258*:1288–1291, 1985.
7. deCampo, T, Aldrete JA: The anesthetic management of the severely burned patient. *Intens Care Med 7*:55-62, 1981.
8. Martyn JAJ, Liu LMP, Szyfelbein SK, Ambalavanar ES, Goudsouzian NG: The neuromuscular effects of pancuronium in burned children. *Anesthesiology 59*:561–564, 1983.
9. Martyn JAJ, Szyfelbein SK, Ali HH, Matteo RS, Savarese JJ: Increased d-tubocurarine requirements following major thermal injury. *Anesthesiology 52*:352–355, 1980.
10. Martyn JAJ, Matteo RS, Szyfelbein SK, Kaplan RF: Unprecedented resistance to neuromuscular blocking effect of metocurine with persistence after complete recovery in a burned patient. *Anesth Analg 61*:614-617, 1982.
11. Martyn JAJ, Goudsouzian NG, Matteo RS, Liu LMP, Szyfelbein SK, Kaplan RF: Metocurine requirements and plasma concentrations in burned paediatric patients. *Br J Anaesth 55*:263-268, 1983.
12. Sawchuk RJ, Rector TS: Drug kinetics in burn patients. *Clin Pharmacokinet 5*:548–556, 1980.
13. Martyn JAH, Matteo RS, Greenblatt DJ, Lebowitz TW, Savarese JJ: Pharmacokinetics of d-tubocurarine in patients with thermal injury. *Anesth Analg 61*:241–246, 1982.
14. Miller RD, Savarese JJ: Pharmacology of muscle relaxants, their agonists and monitoring of neuromuscular function, in *Anesthesia* (Miller RD, ed.). Churchill Livingstone, New York, pp. 487-538, 1981.
15. Leibel WS, Martyn JAJ, Szyfelbein SK, Miller KW: Elevated plasma binding cannot account for the burn related d-tubocurarine hyposensitivity. *Anesthesiology 54*:378–382, 1981.
16. Fambrough DM: Control of acetylcholine receptors in skeletal muscle. *Physiol Rev 59*:165-227, 1979.
17. Almon RR, Appel SH: Cholinergic sites in skeletal muscle I. Denervation effects. *Biochemistry 15*:3662–3667, 1967.

18. Miledi R, Potter LT: The acetylcholine receptor in muscle fibers. *Nature 233*:599–603, 1974.
19. Hartzell HL, Fambrough DM: Acetylcholine receptors distribution and extrajunctional density in rat diaphragm after denervation, correlated with acetylcholine sensitivity. *J Gen Physiol 60*:248–262, 1972.
20. Brenner HR, Sakmann B: Neurotrophic control of channel properties at neuromuscular synapses of rat muscle. *J Physiol 337*:159–171, 1983.
21. Elridge L., Liebold M, Steinbach JH: Alterations in cat skeletal muscle neuromuscular junctions following prolonged activity. *J. Physiol. 313*:529–545, 1981.
22. Moorthy SS, Hilgenberg JC: Resistance to nondepolarizing muscle relaxants in paretic upper extremities of patients with residual hemiplegia. *Anesth Analg 59*:624–627, 1980.
23. Standaert FG: Sites action of muscle relaxants, in *Journal of Clinical Experiences with Norcuron* (Agoston S, Bowman WC, Miller RD, Viby-Morgensen, eds.), Excerpta Medica, Amsterdam, pp. 14–25, 1983.
24. Gronert GA: A possible mechanism for succinylcholine induced hyperkalemia. *Anesthesiology 53*:356, 1980.
25. Standaert FG, Dretchen KL: Cyclic nucleotides in neuromuscular transmission. *Anesth Analg 60*:91–99, 1981.
26. Doll DC, Rosenberg H: Antagonism of neuromuscular blockade by theophylline. *Anesth Analg 58*:139–140, 1979.
27. Eger EI, Smith NT, Cullen DD, et al.: A comparison of cardiovascular effects of halothane, isoflurane, ether and cyclopropane in man. *Anesthesiology 34*:25–41, 1971.
28. Adams AP: Enflurane in clinical practice. *Br J Anaesth 53*: 275, 1981.
29. Eger EI: Isoflurane: A review. *Anesthesiology 55*:559–568, 1981.
30. White PF, Way WL, Trevor AJ: Ketamine: Its pharmacology and therapeutic uses. *56*:119–136, 1982.
31. Lebowitz PW, Ramsey FM, Savarese JJ, et al.: Potentiation of neuromuscular blockade in man produced by combinations of pancuronium and metocurine or pancuronium and d-tubocurarine. *Anesth Analg 59*:604–610, 1980.

32. Satwicz PR, Martyn JAJ, Szyfelbein SK, et al.: Potentiation of neuromuscular blockade using a combination of pancuronium and dimethyltubocurarine. *Br J Anaesth 56*:479–484, 1984.
33. Martyn JJ, Durant J, Szyfelbein SK, Goudsouzian NG: Cardiovascular and neuromuscular pharmacodynamic effect of high dose pancuronium-metocurine combination. *Anesth Analg 60*:252, 1985.
34. Savarese JJ: The new neuromuscular blocking drugs are here. *Anesthesiology 55*:1–3, 1981.

8

Prolonged Apnea Following Succinylcholine Administration

EUGENE J. PANTUCK and CAROL B. PANTUCK
College of Physicians and Surgeons, Columbia University, New York, New York

I. INTRODUCTION

The depolarizing neuromuscular-blocking agent succinylcholine is particularly valuable and very extensively used in the practice of anesthesiology because it is the only skeletal muscle relaxant that has a short duration of action. This short duration of action is primarily the result of its very rapid conversion in plasma by the enzyme plasma cholinesterase to a nearly inactive metabolite. While diffusion from plasma and urinary excretion also play a role in the clearance of succinylcholine from plasma, these factors are normally unimportant relative to hydrolysis of the drug by plasma cholinesterase. Succinylcholine is ordinarily hydrolyzed in plasma at such a rapid rate that only a small fraction of a customary intravenous dose reaches its site of action at the motor end-plates. The action of succinylcholine is terminated by its diffusion away from the end-plates and ultimately back into plasma where it is again exposed to plasma cholinesterase. The larger the concentration of succinylcholine to reach the motor end-plates, the longer the time required for it to diffuse away. Plasma cholinesterase influences the duration of action of a dose of succinylcholine by influencing the concentration of the drug that reaches the motor end-plates and by influencing the length of time during which plasma contains pharmacologically effective levels of drug.

A reduction in the amount or an inhibition of the activity of plasma cholinesterase can be caused by physiological variance, disease, medical treatment, or exposure to environmental pollutants. On occasion, the decrease in plasma cholinesterase activity from such causes can be sufficient to result in a clinically significant prolongation of the effect of succinylcholine. However, the most dramatic increases in the duration of effect of succinylcholine occur in individuals whose plasma contains in place of the normal type of cholinesterase one or a mixture of genetically determined variants which lack or have a markedly diminished capacity for hydrolyzing the drug. In some of these individuals, an intravenous dose of succinylcholine of the size customarily used to facilitate endotracheal intubation will produce neuromuscular blockade lasting several hours rather than the usual 5 to 10 min.

II. PLASMA CHOLINESTERASE—GENERAL PROPERTIES

Plasma cholinesterase (serum cholinesterase, pseudocholinesterase) is a glycoprotein which is synthesized in the liver (1). It is a large molecule consisting of four identical peptide chains, each with a molecular weight of approximately 85,000 daltons (2,3). The physiological role of plasma cholinesterase is not known. The exact mechanism by which plasma cholinesterase catalyzes cleavage of the choline-ester bond has not yet been fully elucidated, nor have the differences between the variants of plasma cholinesterase in amino acid composition that are responsible for the differences in enzymatic activity been established.

III. HYDROLYSIS OF SUCCINYLCHOLINE

Succinylcholine is the dicholine ester of succinic acid (Fig. 1). The enzymatic hydrolysis of succinylcholine by plasma cholinesterase takes place in two steps. First, succinylcholine is hydrolyzed to succinylmonocholine and choline. This occurs very rapidly. Since succinylmonocholine has little neuromuscular-blocking activity, this first step results in the inactivation of succinylcholine. The second step is the hydrolysis of succinylmonocholine to succinic acid and choline. This step proceeds much more slowly than the

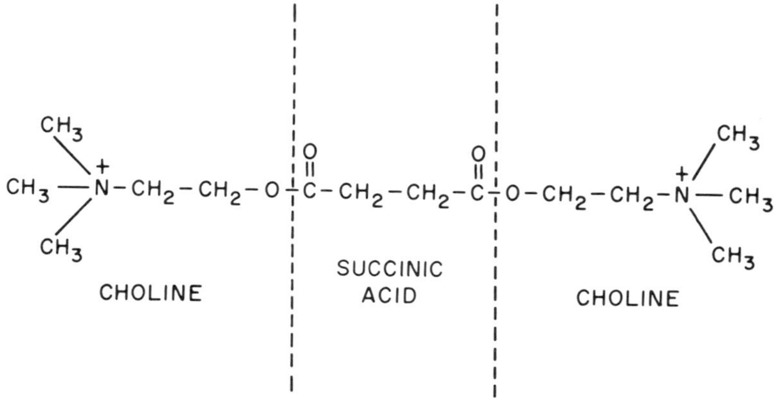

Figure 1 Succinylcholine.

first step. It is catalyzed not only by plasma cholinesterase but also by another esterase which is present in liver.

IV. CHOLINESTERASE ACTIVITY

The cholinesterase activity of an individual's plasma is usually assayed by combining a sample of the plasma with a substance that is hydrolyzed by plasma cholinesterase and measuring the amount of product of the reaction that is released per unit time. If this measurement is carried out to assess the individual's ability to inactivate succinylcholine, then succinylcholine would be the most desirable substrate to use in the assay. However, it is technically very difficult to determine the rate of hydrolysis of succinylcholine and for this reason other substrates such as benzoylcholine and propionylthiocholine are generally used as test substrates to determine plasma cholinesterase activity. There would be no problem in using a test substrate such as benzoylcholine to assess an individual's ability to inactivate succinylcholine if the relationship between the activity of plasma cholinesterase in hydrolyzing the test substrate and the activity of plasma cholinesterase in hydrolyzing succinylcholine were the same for all of the variants of plasma cholinesterase as it is for the normal type of this enzyme. Unfortunately, this has not been found to be the case for any of the test substrates which thus far have been used to measure plasma cholinesterase activity. The problem that arises from using test substrates to assess the ability of the cholinesterase in a sample of plasma to hydrolyze succinylcholine is illustrated by the following example: In plasma that has a cholinesterase activity measured with benzoylcholine that is reduced to 40% of normal as a result of a decrease in amount or inhibition of the normal enzyme, the rate of hydrolysis of succinylcholine will be reduced to a comparable extent. One of the genetically determined abnormal variants of plasma cholinesterase has about 40% of the ability of the normal enzyme to hydrolyze benzoylcholine, but it is incapable of hydrolyzing succinylcholine at clinically occurring concentrations of the drug. In plasma that has a cholinesterase activity measured with benzoylcholine that is 40% of normal as a result of genetically determined replacement of the normal enzyme by this abnormal variant, succinylcholine will not be hydrolyzed at all. Thus, a plasma in which succinylcholine would be hydrolyzed at a substantial rate and a plasma in which succinylcholine would not be hydrolyzed at all could both have a cholinesterase activity measured with benzoylcholine of 40% of normal. To establish what the cholinesterase activity of a sample of plasma as measured with a test substrate means with respect to the ability of the cholinesterase in the plasma to hydrolyze succinylcholine, it is also necessary to ascertain the type of cholinesterase present in the plasma. As will be discussed later, this is accomplished through the use of differential inhibitors of the plasma cholinesterase variants.

V. PLASMA CHOLINESTERASE ACTIVITY AND RESPONSE TO SUCCINYLCHOLINE

Viby-Mogensen has studied response to succinylcholine in a large series of patients with widely varying levels of the normal type of plasma cholinesterase (4). In patients who have a normal level of activity of the normal type of plasma cholinesterase, an intravenous dose of succinylcholine of 1 mg/kg produces approximately 6 min of total apnea and approximately 10 min of neuromuscular blockade (recovery defined as return of first twitch in

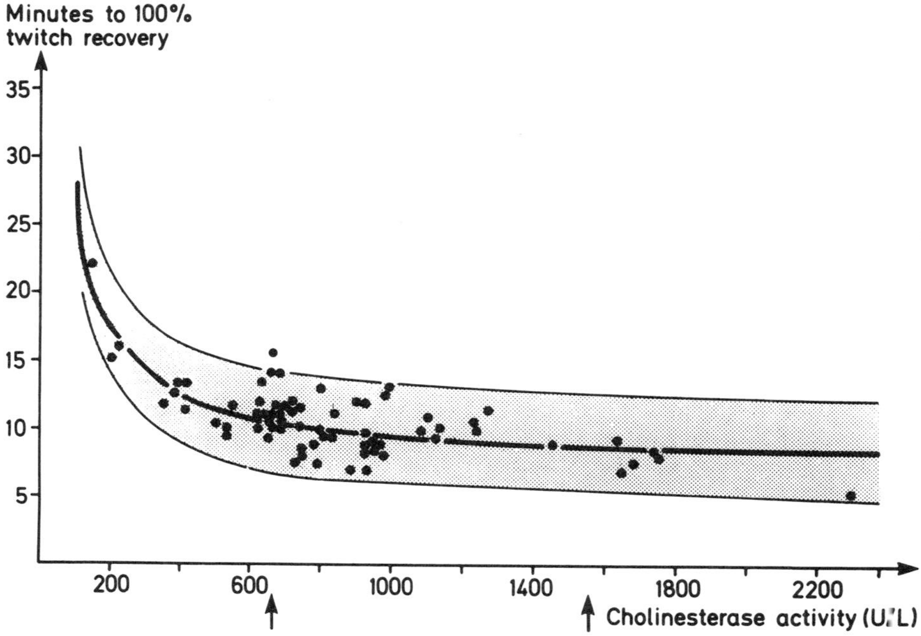

Figure 2 Relationship between enzymatic activity and time to recovery of 100% twitch height following administration of succinylcholine, 1 mg/kg i.v., to 70 patients with the normal plasma cholinesterase genotype. The fitted regression line and 95% prediction region are given. Arrows indicate the normal range of plasma cholinesterase activity. (From Ref. 4, used with permission.)

response to train-of-four stimulation to control level). The relationship between plasma cholinesterase activity and time to recovery from neuromuscular block following the administration of succinylcholine, 1 mg/kg i.v., in patients with the normal type of enzyme is shown in Figure 2. The mean level of plasma cholinesterase activity for the patients whose activity fell within the normal range was approximately 900 U/L. Esterase activity of 400-500 U/L, approximately 50% of mean normal, resulted in only a small increase in mean duration of neuromuscular blockade. Even esterase activity as low as 150 U/L resulted in only a moderate prolongation in recovery time.

VI. PLASMA CHOLINESTERASE DEFICIENCY—NORMAL ENZYME

A. Causes

There are a large number of causes of reduced activity of the normal plasma cholinesterase enzyme (5,6). For the most part, these causes of reduced cholinesterase activity do not produce enough of a decrease to impair the metabolism of succinylcholine sufficiently to result in more than a slight increase in duration of its action. Clinically significant prolonged response to succinylcholine has been reported to have occurred in patients with cholinesterase activity reduced as a result of pregnancy (7-12), liver disease (13,14), cancer (14), treatment with cyclophosphamide (14-16), treatment with phenelzine (17), treatment with echothiophate iodide eye drops (14,18-22), treatment with plasmapheresis (23,24), and exposure to organophosphate insecticides (25).

1. Pregnancy

A reduction in plasma cholinesterase activity occurs during the first trimester of pregnancy, probably as a result of reduced synthesis of the enzyme, and persists into the early postpartum period (10,11,26-30). The size of the decrease is ordinarily small, averaging about 25-30% (10,11,26-30), but individuals with plasma cholinesterase activity as low as 20-30% of mean normal have been observed (10,30).

2. Liver Disease

In prolonged severe liver disease, marked reduction of plasma cholinesterase activity is common (13,31,32). Decreases of more than 75% can occur (13,14). The decrease in plasma cholinesterase activity is the result of reduced synthesis of the enzyme.

3. Cancer

Reduced plasma cholinesterase activity is common in patients with malignant tumors, particularly those of the genitourinary tract, gastrointestinal tract, and lung (33). The mechanism of the reduction is not clear. The size of the decrease is usually modest, but it can be substantial, especially in patients with bronchogenic carcinoma (33). Levels of plasma cholinesterase activity <25% of mean normal have been observed (14).

4. Phenelzine

Phenelzine is a monoamine oxidase inhibitor that is used in the treatment of severe mental depression. Marked reduction in plasma cholinesterase activity occurs in some patients receiving this drug (17). A decrease caused by phenelzine in plasma cholinesterase activity of >90% has been observed (17). The mechanism by which phenelzine produces a decrease in plasma cholinesterase activity is not known.

5. Cyclophosphamide

The cytotoxic drug cyclophosphamide which is used in the treatment of cancer, is an organophosphate compound that is a potent, long-acting inhibitor of plasma cholinesterase (34). Although usually less, reduction in plasma cholinesterase activity of 70% has been seen in patients receiving this drug (16,34,35).

6. Echothiophate Iodide

Echothiophate iodide is an organophosphate compound which is a potent, long-acting inhibitor of plasma cholinesterase. It is used in the form of eyedrops in the treatment of glaucoma. There is systemic absorption sufficient to produce marked decreases in plasma cholinesterase activity in patients who are treated with these eyedrops for a prolonged period of time (36,37). A decrease in plasma cholinesterase activity of about 70% is typical in such patients, but decreases of >95% have been observed (37).

7. Plasmapheresis

Plasmapheresis is a technique for removing circulating antibodies from patients which is used in the management of autoimmune disorders and in the control of Rh incompatibility in pregnancy. In this procedure, plasma is removed and is replaced with a colloid or crystalloid solution, resulting in a decrease in plasma cholinesterase concentration. A single 4-L plasma exchange results in a 50–70% decrease in plasma cholinesterase activity (38), and repeated daily plasma exchange can result in virtually the total depletion of plasma cholinesterase (38,39).

8. Organophosphate Insecticides

Organophosphate insecticides are long-acting inhibitors of plasma cholinesterase. Poisoning with organophosphate insecticides is common in agricultural areas. Essentially total inhibition of plasma cholinesterase activity can occur in individuals exposed to these compounds (25).

B. Response to Succinylcholine

Reference to Figure 2 makes it clear that only an extremely large decrease in plasma cholinesterase activity will result in more than a small increase in duration of response to an ordinary clinical dose of succinylcholine. Nevertheless, there are numerous reports of patients with modest decreases in plasma cholinesterase activity resulting from such causes as pregnancy having markedly prolonged apnea following ordinary doses of succinylcholine. In considering these reports, it should be borne in mind that in few, if any, has prolonged neuromuscular blockade been documented by the use of a nerve stimulator and that in anesthetized patients who have received succinylcholine there are causes of prolonged apnea other than prolonged response to that drug. Also, as will be discussed later, there is evidence for the existence of genetically determined abnormal variants of plasma cholinesterase that are incapable of metabolizing succinylcholine but appear normal in type when tested with the biochemical methods currently in use. If such variants do exist, it is possible that in a patient who presents an obvious reason, such as pregnancy, for a decreased level of normal enzyme, there could be an abnormal variant of the enzyme that is not recognized instead of the normal enzyme.

VII. PLASMA CHOLINESTERASE DEFICIENCY—ABNORMAL ENZYME VARIANTS

A. Dibucaine-Resistant Variant

Kalow and his associates were the first to demonstrate clearly that prolonged response to succinylcholine could result not only from a decreased amount of the usual type of plasma cholinesterase, but also from replacement of this enzyme by an abnormal variant (40,41). They found in the plasma of individuals who had experienced markedly prolonged response to succinylcholine, cholinesterase that was qualitatively different from the usual enzyme in that it was totally unable to hydrolyze succinylcholine at the concentrations of this drug that occur in blood under clinical circumstances and in that it was far more resistant to inhibition by the local anesthetic dibucaine (40,42). They used this difference between the normal and abnormal variants in resistance to inhibition by dibucaine as the basis of a test to distinguish between them (40). Dibucaine, as used in this test, inhibits the hydrolysis of benzoylcholine by normal plasma cholinesterase by 70% or more, whereas it inhibits hydrolysis by the abnormal variant by 30% or less. The term dibucaine number was applied to the percentage of inhibition of activity of plasma cholinesterase in hydrolyzing benzoylcholine produced by dibucaine under the standardized test conditions. Therefore, plasma containing normal cholinesterase would receive a dibucaine number of ≥ 70, and plasma containing the abnormal variant would receive a dibucaine number of ≤ 30.

The manner in which the dibucaine test distinguishes individuals whose plasma contains the normal type of cholinesterase from individuals whose plasma contains the abnormal variant is illustrated in Figure 3. The dibucaine number identifies the plasma

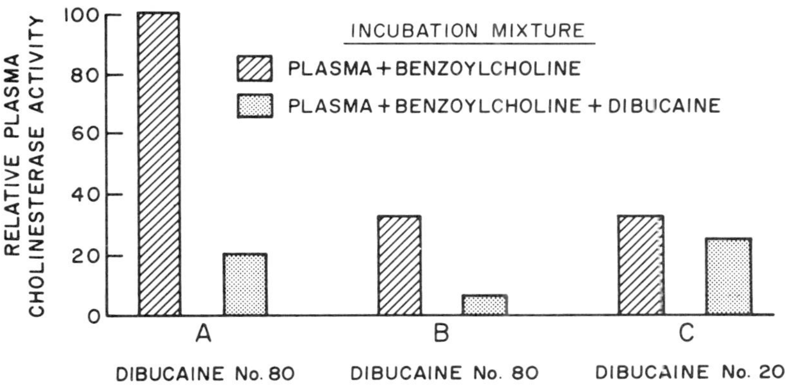

Figure 3 Use of dibucaine test to distinguish between normal plasma cholinesterase and the dibucaine-resistant variant. A, Patient with normal amount of normal type of plasma cholinesterase. B, Patient with decreased amount of normal type of plasma cholinesterase. C, Patient with dibucaine-resistant variant of plasma cholinesterase. [From Pantuck EJ, Pantuck CB: Cholinesterases and anticholinesterases, in *Muscle Relaxants* (Katz RL, ed.), Excerpta Medica, Elsevier, Amsterdam, pp. 143-162, 1975, used with permission.]

with the abnormal variant of plasma cholinesterase because the percent inhibition produced by dibucaine is dependent only on the type of plasma cholinesterase present and is independent of the absolute activity of the enzyme in hydrolyzing benzoylcholine. The dibucaine test, by identifying the type of cholinesterase present in plasma, makes it possible to assess what the cholinesterase activity measured with a test substrate such as benzoylcholine means with respect to the ability of the cholinesterase in the plasma to hydrolyze succinylcholine. In Figure 3, patients B and C both have a plasma cholinesterase activity of 33% of normal, but patient B will have a considerable ability to hydrolyze succinylcholine and will exhibit only a small increase in response to this drug, whereas patient C will have no ability to hydrolyze succinylcholine and will have a large increase in response to the drug.

Kalow and his colleagues found that the dibucaine test separated individuals into three groups with dibucaine numbers, respectively, of ⩾70, ⩽30, and between 40 and 70 (40,43). Their data indicated that the type of cholinesterase contained in an individual's plasma is determined by two allelic, autosomal, codominant genes (43). (Allelic, the genes for the normal and abnormal enzymes occur at the same locus, and therefore only one or the other can be present on each one of the appropriate pair of chomosomes; autosomal, the gene does not occur on a sex chromosome, and therefore its transmission is not sex linked; codominant, each gene controls the production of its particular enzyme unaffected by the corresponding gene on the other chromosome.) Thus, an individual with a dibucaine number of ⩾70 would be a homozygote with two genes for the normal enzyme and plasma containing only the normal enzyme. An individual with a dibucaine number of ⩽30 would be a homozygote with two genes for the abnormal variant of the enzyme and plasma containing only the abnormal variant. An individual with a dibucaine number between 40 and 70 would be a heterozygote with one gene for the normal enzyme, one gene for the abnormal variant, and plasma containing a mixture of the two types of cholinesterase.

Surveys in a number of European and American caucasian populations have found the frequency of occurrence of heterozygotes for the normal and dibucaine-resistant genes to be about one in 25, and the frequency of occurrence of homozygotes for the dibucaine-resistant gene to be about one in 2500 (44,45). The dibucaine-resistant gene is rare in blacks and orientals (44-46).

In patients heterozygous for the normal and dibucaine-resistant genes, duration of apnea and time of recovery from neuromuscular block (return of first twitch in the response to train-of-four stimulation to 90% of control level) following the administration of succinylcholine, 1 mg/kg i.v., were found to be approximately 10 and 15 min, respectively (47). In patients homozygous for the dibucaine-resistant gene, recovery from neuromuscular block following administration of succinylcholine, 1 mg/kg i.v., was found to require approximately 2.5-3.5 hr (48).

B. Fluoride-Resistant Variant

Harris and Whittaker found that sodium fluoride, like dibucaine, is a differential inhibitor of the normal and dibucaine-resistant variants of plasma cholinesterase (49). They applied the term fluoride number to the percentage of inhibition of activity of plasma cholinesterase in hydrolyzing benzoylcholine produced by sodium fluoride under standardized conditions. For the most part, they found a good correlation between the dibucaine number and the fluoride number, but a few individuals classified by the dibucaine number as homozygotes for the normal gene or as heterozygotes for the normal and dibucaine-resistant genes had lower fluoride numbers than usually found in individuals in their respective categories. These discrepancies led them to the recognition of a variant of plasma cholinesterase markedly resistant to inhibition by sodium fluoride but, unlike the dibucaine-resistant variant, only slightly resistant to inhibition by dibucaine. They found the production of this fluoride-resistant variant of plasma cholinesterase to be controlled by a gene allelic to the normal and dibucaine-resistant cholinesterase genes.

The fluoride-resistant gene is extremely rare (45), though it has been found with a high frequency in a Punjabi population in India (50).

The fluoride-resistant variant of plasma cholinesterase has some ability, though less than normal, to hydrolyze succinylcholine. Evidence obtained from patients heterozygous for the fluoride-resistant gene suggests that in patients homozygous for the gene, the duration of neuromuscular block following an ordinary clinical dose of succinylcholine is likely to be increased in the order of magnitude of two- to threefold (47,51).

C. Silent Variants

The discovery of healthy individuals whose plasma totally lacked cholinesterase activity (52,53) led to the recognition of two or possibly more variants of plasma cholinesterase that lacked the necessary structure to effectively hydrolyze the choline-ester bond (52–58). The production of these variants has been found to be controlled by genes, called silent genes, which are allelic to the normal, dibucaine-resistant, and fluoride-resistant cholinesterase genes (54,59). Since there is no clinical significance to any small differences that may exist in the ability of these variants to hydrolyze succinylcholine, the silent genes will be treated in this chapter as if they were a single entity.

The silent gene for plasma cholinesterase is extremely rare (45), though it has been found with a high frequency in several Alaskan Eskimo groups (54,58,60), some caucasian South Africans (61), and in a Vysyas caste group in India (62).

The limited evidence available suggests that homozygotes for the silent gene react to succinylcholine similarly to homozygotes for the dibucaine-resistant gene (48,63).

D. Characteristics of Plasma Cholinesterase Genotypes

The four allelic genes for plasma cholinesterase, the normal, dibucaine-resistant, fluoride-resistant, and silent, can combine to form 10 genotypes. Biochemical characteristics of the genotypes are presented in Table 1, and information on the response to succinylcholine of patients with the various genotypes is presented in Tables 1 and 2. In these tables, Motulsky's system of nomenclature (64) is used to designate the genotypes. In this system, the locus of the genes is designated E_1 (E for esterase). The gene designated E_1^u produces the most common (usual) form of cholinesterase. The gene designated E_1^a produces the dibucaine-resistant (originally called atypical) variant; E_1^f produces the fluoride-resistant variant; and E_1^s is actually two or more genes (called silent genes because the first identified was initially thought to cause the production of no enzyme) producing variants with little or no activity.

E. Unrecognized Variants

Published studies of cholinesterase genotype distribution in patients who had prolonged apnea following the administration of succinylcholine have all reported a substantial (13–51%) incidence of individuals who have normal plasma cholinesterase activity and dibucaine and fluoride numbers characteristic of the normal genotype (5,14,65–71). These findings suggest the possibility that there may be variants of plasma cholinesterase that have

Table 1 Characteristics of Genotypes Resulting from Four Alleles at the E_1 Locus

Genotype	Relative mean enzymatic activity with benzoylcholine substrate[a]	Typical dibucaine number	Typical fluoride number	Response to succinylcholine
$E_1^u E_1^u$	100	80	60	Normal
$E_1^a E_1^a$	43	20	20	Very prolonged
$E_1^f E_1^f$	74	65	35	Moderately prolonged
$E_1^s E_1^s$	0 or Slight	—	—	Very prolonged
$E_1^u E_1^a$	77	60	50	Slightly prolonged
$E_1^u E_1^f$	86	75	50	Slightly prolonged
$E_1^u E_1^s$	50	80	60	Slightly prolonged
$E_1^a E_1^f$	59	50	50	Moderately prolonged
$E_1^a E_1^s$	22	20	20	Very prolonged
$E_1^f E_1^s$	37	65	35	Moderately prolonged

[a]From Ref. 5.

Table 2 Duration of Apnea and Time to Recovery From Neuromuscular Blockade Following Intravenous Administration of Succinylcholine (1 mg/kg) in Patients with Genotypes Resulting from Four Alleles at the E_1 Locus

Genotype	No. patients	Duration of apnea (min)		Recovery of first twitch in train-of-four response to 90% of control height (min)		Recovery of train-of-four ratio to 0.7 (min)	
		Mean	Range	Mean	Range	Mean	Range
$E_1^uE_1^u$	41[a]	5.8	4.0–9.0	9.3	6.0–13.0		
$E_1^aE_1^a$	2[b]					144	137–152
$E_1^fE_1^f$	—						
$E_1^sE_1^s$	1[c]					140	
$E_1^uE_1^a$	28[d]	9.5	5.0–16.0	14.6	8.0–22.0		
$E_1^uE_1^f$	3[d]	7.3	7.0–8.0	12.0	11.0–13.0		
$E_1^uE_1^s$	8[d]	8.7	4.0–12.0	12.4	7.5–18.0		
$E_1^aE_1^f$	3[d]	24.0	23.0–26.0	29.5	29.0–30.0		
$E_1^aE_1^s$	—						
$E_1^fE_1^s$	1[d]	27.0		30.0			

[a]From Ref. 4.
[b]From Ref. 48.
[c]From Ref. 63.
[d]From Ref. 47.

an impaired ability to metabolize succinylcholine, but are not identified by the conventional tests that are currently employed. Using a method which employs succinylcholine itself as substrate, Goedde and Agarwal found that sera from seven of 36 patients who had a prolonged apnea following succinylcholine administration, and who had previously been classified as having normal cholinesterase activity and genotype, had no activity in hydrolyzing this relaxant (72).

It seems likely that many of the patients who have been reported to have had prolonged apnea after receiving succinylcholine and to have normal cholinesterase activity and type have had the prolonged apnea for reasons other than abnormal response to the relaxant. Sixty-three (28%) of 225 patients reported to the Danish Cholinesterase Research Unit for prolonged apnea resulting from succinylcholine were found to have normal cholinesterase activity and to be of normal genotype (14). On careful review, a reason for prolonged apnea other than abnormal response to succinylcholine, such as overdosage with central respiratory depressant drugs, was identified in 34 of these cases (14). Seven of the remaining 29 patients were subsequently anesthetized again. They were monitored with a nerve stimulator, and all reacted normally to succinylcholine (6).

VIII. MANAGEMENT OF PROLONGED RESPONSE TO SUCCINYLCHOLINE

It should not be assumed that prolonged apnea following administration of succinylcholine is necessarily due to an abnormal response to that drug. It may be due to other causes such as overdosage with central respiratory depressant drugs or hyperventilation. If prolonged response to succinylcholine is suspected of being the cause of the prolonged apnea, a nerve stimulator should be used to determine whether the apnea is accompanied by neuromuscular blockade. Absence of neuromuscular blockade will establish that the apnea is not due to succinylcholine. If the dose of succinylcholine has been modest and no other relaxants have been used, then the presence of neuromuscular blockade will establish that the prolonged apnea has resulted from an abnormal response to succinylcholine.

The only necessary treatment for prolonged response to succinylcholine is adequate pulmonary ventilation until the return of normal neuromuscular function.

An ordinary intravenous dose of succinylcholine normally produces a neuromuscular block of the depolarizing type. Prolonged exposure of the motor end-plates to large concentrations of succinylcholine causes a change in the character of the block to nondepolarizing (73-76). The depolarizing block is called phase I block, and the nondepolarizing block phase II block. Conversion of the block from phase I to phase II occurs following the administration of an ordinary dose of succinylcholine in patients who have a substantial impairment in their ability to metabolize this drug (6,47,48,51,63,75,77).

A phase II block can be antagonized by anticholinesterases (48,76,78). The question, therefore, exists as to whether in the management of prolonged response to succinylcholine, anticholinesterases can be administered when the block has become phase II in character to reduce recovery time. Unfortunately, the outcome of such treatment can be potentiation rather than antagonism of the effects of succinylcholine, and is dependent on factors that cannot be evaluated easily (48,75-77). Although anticholinesterases will antagonize a phase II block (48,76,78), they will potentiate a phase I block (75). As long as a pharmacologically effective level of succinylcholine remains in the plasma, a component of phase I block will persist and will be potentiated by the administration of an anticholinesterase (48,76). In the presence of a well-established phase II block, the extent to which a phase I block may also be present cannot clearly be identified by the use of a nerve stimulator. Following the intravenous administration of 1 mg/kg of succinylcholine to individuals incapable of metabolizing this drug, a pharmacologically effective level can persist in plasma for more than 90 min (48).

Termination of prolonged succinylcholine neuromuscular block can be reliably accelerated by first administering human plasma cholinesterase to hydrolyze succinylcholine, thereby ending the phase I component of the block, and then administering an anticholinesterase to terminate the phase II component of the block (48). A purified preparation of human cholinesterase is available in Europe but not in North America. Cholinesterase activity is preserved in bank blood (79-81), so that transfusion of blood or plasma can be used to terminate the phase I component of the block. However, when the risks of transfusion are weighed against the risks of ventilatory support, transfusion will rarely be justifiable.

Patients who have a prolonged response to succinylcholine should be tested for plasma cholinesterase activity and type. Patients found to be of genotypes that place them at risk of clinically significant prolonged response to succinylcholine should be told to present this information to anesthesiologists who care for them. Relatives of such individuals should also be tested for plasma cholinesterase activity and type and similarly advised.

REFERENCES

1. Svensmark O: Molecular properties of cholinesterases. *Acta Physiol Scand 64*(Suppl 245):1-74, 1965.
2. Lockridge O, Eckerson HW, La Du BN: Interchain disulfide bonds and subunit organization in human serum cholinesterase. *J Biol Chem 254*:8324-8330, 1979.
3. Haupt H, Heide K, Zwisler O, Schwick HG: Isolierung und physikalisch-chemische Charakterisierung der Cholinesterase aus Humanserum. *Blut 14*:65-75, 1966.
4. Viby-Mogensen J: Correlation of succinylcholine duration of action with plasma cholinesterase activity in subjects with the genotypically normal enzyme. *Anesthesiology 53*:517-520, 1980.
5. Whittaker M: Plasma cholinesterase variants and the anaesthetist. *Anaesthesia 35*:174-197, 1980.
6. Viby-Mogensen J: Cholinesterase and succinylcholine. *Dan Med Bull 30*:129-150, 1983.
7. Macdonald AG, Graham IH: Suxamethonium apnoea in a pregnant patient. *Br J Anaesth 40*:711-712, 1968.
8. Wildsmith JAW: Serum cholinesterase, pregnancy and suxamethonium. *Anaesthesia 27*:90-91, 1972.
9. Weissman DB, Ehrenwerth J: Prolonged neuromuscular blockade in a parturient associated with succinylcholine. *Anesth Analg 62*:444-446, 1983.

10. Robertson GS: Serum cholinesterase deficiency II: Pregnancy. *Br J Anaesth 38*:361–369, 1966.
11. Shnider SM: Serum cholinesterase activity during pregnancy, labor and the puerperium. *Anesthesiology 26*:335–339, 1965.
12. Ravindran RS, Cummins DF, Pantazias KL, Strausburg BJ, Baenziger JC: Unusual aspects of low levels of pseudocholinesterase in a pregnant patient. *Anesth Analg 61*:953–955, 1982.
13. Foldes FF, Rendell-Baker L, Birch JH: Causes and prevention of prolonged apnea with succinylcholine. *Anesth Analg 35*: 609-633, 1956.
14. Viby-Mogensen J, Hanel HK: Prolonged apnoea after suxamethonium. An analysis of the first 225 cases reported to the Danish Cholinesterase Research Unit. *Acta Anaesthesiol Scand 22*:371–380, 1978.
15. Gurman GM: Prolonged apnea after succinylcholine in a patient treated with cytostatics for cancer. *Anesth Analg 51*: 761–765, 1972.
16. Walker IR, Zapf PW, Mackay IR: Cyclophosphamide, cholinesterase and anaesthesia. *Aust NZ J Med 2*:247–251, 1972.
17. Bodley PO, Halwax K, Potts L: Low serum pseudocholinesterase levels complicating treatment with phenelzine. *Br Med J 3*:510–512, 1969.
18. Pantuck EJ: Ecothiopate iodide eye drops and prolonged response to suxamethonium. *Br J Anaesth 38*:406–407, 1966.
19. Gesztes T: Prolonged apnoea after suxamethonium injection associated with eye drops containing an anticholinesterase agent. *Br J Anaesth 38*:408–410, 1966.
20. Packman PM, Meyer DA, Verdun RM: Hazards of succinylcholine administration during electrotherapy. *Arch Gen Psychiatry 35*:1137–1141, 1978.
21. Cavallaro RJ, Krumperman LW, Kugler F: Effect of echothiophate therapy on the metabolism of succinylcholine in man. *Anesth Analg 47*:570–574, 1968.
22. Chessen DH, Geha DG, Salzman C: ECT, glaucoma and prolonged apnea. *Dis Nerv Syst 35*:152–153, 1974.
23. Lumley J: Prolongation of suxamethonium following plasma exchange. *Br J Anaesth 52*:1149–1150, 1980.

24. Evans RT, Macdonald R, Robinson A: Suxamethonium apnoea associated with plasmapheresis. *Anaesthesia 35*: 198-201, 1980.
25. Weis OF, Muller FO, Lyell H, Badenhorst CH, van Niekerk P: Materno-fetal cholinesterase inhibitor poisoning. *Anesth Analg 62*:233-235, 1983.
26. Blitt CD, Petty WC, Alberterst EE, Wright BJ: Correlation of plasma cholinesterase activity and duration of action of succinylcholine during pregnancy. *Anesth Analg 56*:78-83, 1977.
27. Howard JK, East NJ, Chaney JL: Plasma cholinesterase activity in early pregnancy. *Arch Environ Health 33*:277-279, 1978.
28. Ganga CC, Heyduk JV, Marx GF, Sklar GS: A comparison of the response to suxamethonium in post-partum and gynaecological patients. *Anaesthesia 37*:903-906, 1982.
29. Evans RT, Wroe JM: Plasma cholinesterase changes during pregnancy. Their interpretation as a cause of suxamethonium-induced apnoea. *Anaesthesia 35*:651-654, 1980.
30. Hazel B, Monier D: Human serum cholinesterase: Variations during pregnancy and post-partum. *Can Anaesth Soc J 18*: 272-277, 1971.
31. McArdle B: The serum cholinesterase in jaundice and diseases of the liver. *Q J Med 9*:107-127, 1940.
32. Singh DS, Shukla PK, Gupta JP, Dube B: Serum cholinesterase in hepatic disorders. *J Indian Med Assoc 66*:49-51, 1976.
33. Kaniaris P, Fassoulaki A, Liarmakopoulou K, Dermitzakis E: Serum cholinesterase levels in patients with cancer. *Anesth Analg 58*:82-84, 1979.
34. Zsigmond EK, Robins G: The effect of a series of anti-cancer drugs on plasma cholinesterase activity. *Can Anaesth Soc J 19*:75-82, 1972.
35. Mone JG, Mathie WE: Qualitative and quantitative defects of pseudocholinesterase activity. *Anaesthesia 22*:55-68, 1967.
36. McGavin DDM: Depressed levels of serum-pseudocholinesterase with ecothiophate-iodide eyedrops. *Lancet 2*:272-273, 1965.

37. de Roetth A, Jr, Dettbarn W-D, Rosenberg P, Wilensky JG, Wong A: Effect of phospholine iodide on blood cholinesterase levels of normal and glaucoma subjects. *Am J Ophthalmol 59*:586-592, 1965.
38. Wood GJ, Hall GM: Plasmapheresis and plasma cholinesterase. *Br J Anaesth 50*:945-949, 1978.
39. Paterson JL, Walsh ES, Hall GM: Progressive depletion of plasma cholinesterase during daily plasma exchange. *Br Med J 2*:580, 1979.
40. Kalow W, Genest K: A method for the detection of atypical forms of human serum cholinesterase. Determination of dibucaine numbers. *Can J Biochem Physiol 35*:339-346, 1957.
41. Kalow W, Gunn DR: The relation between dose of succinylcholine and duration of apnea in man. *J Pharmacol Exp Ther 120*:203-214, 1957.
42. Kalow W: The distribution, destruction and elimination of muscle relaxants. *Anesthesiology 20*:505-518, 1959.
43. Kalow W, Staron N: On distribution and inheritance of atypical forms of human serum cholinesterase, as indicated by dibucaine numbers. *Can J Biochem Physiol 35*:1305-1317, 1957.
44. Lubin AH, Garry PJ, Owen GM: Sex and population differences in the incidence of a plasma cholinesterase variant. *Science 173*:161-164, 1971.
45. Steegmuller H: On the geographical distribution of pseudocholinesterase variants. *Humangenetik 26*:167-185, 1975.
46. Motulsky AG, Morrow A: Atypical cholinesterase gene E_1^a. Rarity in negroes and most orientals. *Science 159*:202, 1968.
47. Viby-Mogensen J: Succinylcholine neuromuscular blockade in subjects heterozygous for abnormal plasma cholinesterase. *Anesthesiology 55*:231-235, 1981.
48. Viby-Mogensen J: Succinylcholine neuromuscular blockade in subjects homozygous for atypical plasma cholinesterase. *Anesthesiology 55*:429-434, 1981.
49. Harris H, Whittaker M: Differential inhibition of human serum cholinesterase with fluoride. Recognition of two new phenotypes. *Nature 191*:496-498, 1961.

50. Singh S, Amma MKP, Sareen KN, Goedde HW: A study of the pseudocholinesterase polymorphism among a Punjabi population. *Hum Hered 21*:388-393, 1971.
51. Viby-Mogensen J, Hanel HK: Increased sensitivity to succinylcholine in a patient heterozygous for the silent and the fluoride-resistant gene. *Anesth Analg 57*:422-427, 1978.
52. Liddell J, Lehmann H, Silk E: A "silent" pseudocholinesterase gene. *Nature 193*:561-562, 1962.
53. Hart SM, Mitchell JV: Suxamethonium in the absence of pseudocholinesterase. *Br J Anaesth 34*:207-209, 1962.
54. Scott EM: Inheritance of two types of deficiency of human serum cholinesterase. *Ann Hum Genet 37*:139-143, 1973.
55. Lubin AH, Garry PJ, Owen GM, Prince LC, and Dietz AA: Further variation of the "silent" cholinesterase gene. *Biochem Med 8*:160-165, 1973.
56. LaMotta RV, Woronick CL: Molecular heterogeneity of human serum cholinesterase. *Clin Chem 17*:135-144, 1971.
57. Rubinstein HM, Dietz AA, Hodges LK, Lubrano T, Czebotar V: Silent cholinesterase gene: Variations in the properties of serum enzyme in apparent homozygotes. *J Clin Invest 49*: 479-486, 1970.
58. Scott EM, Wright RC: A third type of serum cholinesterase deficiency in Eskimos. *Am J Hum Genet 28*:253-256, 1976.
59. Simpson NE, Kalow W: The "silent" gene for serum cholinesterase. *Am J Hum Genet 16*:180-188, 1964.
60. Gutsche BB, Scott EM, Wright RC: Hereditary deficiency of pseudocholinesterase in Eskimos. *Nature 215*:322-323, 1967.
61. Pannall PR, Potgieter GM, Raubenheimer MM: Plasma cholinesterase variants—An unexpectedly high incidence of the silent allele. *S Afr Med J 50*:304-306, 1976.
62. Rao PR, Gopalam KB: High incidence of the silent allele at cholinesterase locus 1 in Vysyas of Andhra Pradesh (S. India). *Hum Genet 52*:139-141, 1979.
63. Oshita S, Sari A, Fujii S, Yonei A: Prolonged neuromuscular blockade following succinylcholine in a patient homozygous for the silent gene. *Anesthesiology 59*:71-73, 1983.
64. Motulsky AG: Pharmacogenetics. *Prog Med Genet 3*:49-74, 1964.

65. Kalow W: Contribution of hereditary factors to the response to drugs. *Fed Proc 24*:1259–1265, 1965.
66. Thompson JC, Whittacker M: A study of the pseudocholinesterase in 78 cases of apnoea following suxamethonium. *Acta Genet 16*:209–222, 1966.
67. Lehmann H, Liddell J: Human cholinesterase (pseudocholinesterase): Genetic variants and their recognition. *Br J Anaesth 41*:235–244, 1969.
68. Whittaker M, Vickers MD: Initial experiences with the Cholinesterase Research Unit. *Br J Anaesth 42*:1016–1020, 1970.
69. Berry M and Whittaker M: Incidence of suxamethonium apnoea in patients undergoing E.C.T. *Br J Anaesth 47*:1195–1197, 1975.
70. Bauld HW, Gibson PF, Jebson PJ, Brown SS: Aetiology of prolonged apnoea after suxamethonium. *Br J Anaesth 46*: 273–281, 1974.
71. Goedde HW, Munsch H, Benkmann H-G, Scholler KL: Succinyldicholin-Empfindlichkeit als Folge genetisch bedingter Serumcholinesterasevarianten. *Prakt Anaesth 11*: 339–346, 1976.
72. Goedde HW, Agarwal DP: Pseudocholinesterase variation. *Hum Genet 1*(Suppl):45–55, 1978.
73. Brennan HJ: Dual action of suxamethonium chloride. *Br J Anaesth 28*:159–168, 1956.
74. Lee C: Dose-relationships of phase II, tachyphylaxis, and train-of-four fade in suxamethonium-induced dual neuromuscular block in man. *Br J Anaesth 47*:841–845, 1975.
75. Baraka A: Suxamethonium-neostigmine interaction in patients with normal or atypical cholinesterase. *Br J Anaesth 49*:479–484, 1977.
76. Gissen AJ, Katz RL, Karis JH, Papper EM: Neuromuscular block in man during prolonged arterial infusion with succinylcholine. *Anesthesiology 27*:242–249, 1966.
77. Vickers MDA: The mismanagement of suxamethonium apnoea. *Br J Anaesth 35*:260–268, 1963.
78. Donati F, and Bevan DR: Antagonism of phase II succinylcholine block by neostigmine. *Anesth Analg 64*:773–776, 1985.

79. Lanks KW, Sklar GS: Stability of pseudocholinesterase in stored blood. *Anesthesiology 44*:428-430, 1976.
80. Schuh FT: Pseudocholinesterase activity of human whole blood, bank blood and blood protein solutions. *Anaesthetist 24*:103-106, 1975.
81. Epstein HM, Jarzemsky D, Zuckerman L, Vagher P: Plasma cholinesterase activity in bank blood. *Anesth Analg 59*: 211-214, 1980.

Index

Q

R

S

T

U

V